I0022820

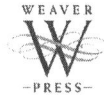

WEAVER
W
—PRESS—

Kwela
B·O·O·K·S

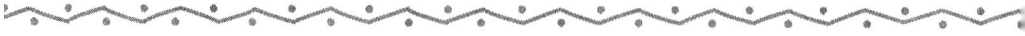

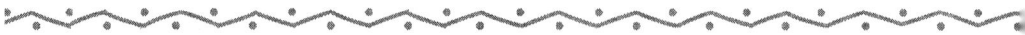

ABC

*of all the questions
we never dare to ask*

KWELA BOOKS & WEAVER PRESS

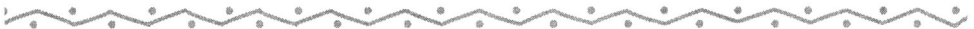

Acknowledgements

The publishers wish to thank the following people for their indispensible contribution to this book. In Zimbabwe:

Inam Chitsike, Tsitsi Dangarembizi, Keith Goddard, Barbara Kaim, Naira Khan, Vivienne Kernhohan, Caroline Maposhure, Betty Mukiibi, Mary Ndlovu, Innocentia Nyoni, Shelia Piano, Taurai Piano, Sunanda Ray and Olivia Zvedi.

In South Africa:

Ricki Fransman, Ann Gordon, Roro Makubalo, Sebi Oliphant, Naeema Parker and Monica Robertson of Childline; Jacqui Gallinetti at the Community Law Centre, University of the Western Cape; E K M Dido and Liesel Dietmann.

Kwela Books
40 Heerengracht, Cape Town 8001;
P.O. Box 6525, Roggebaai 8012
http://www.kwela.com

Weaver Press
Box 1922, Avondale
Harare
http://www.weaverpresszimbabwe.com

Illustrations by Stefan van der Merwe
Cover design and typography by Nazli Jacobs
Set in Gill Sans Schoolbook
Printed and bound by Paarl Print, Oosterland Street, Paarl, South Africa

First edition, first printing 2003
South Africa   ISBN 0-7957-0154-3
Zimbabwe   ISBN 1 77922 023 5

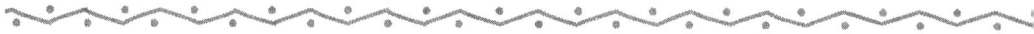

Foreword

For many generations adolescents have been appealing to adults for a break in the silence regarding life expectancies and experiences. Adults in turn have shied away and by not providing sufficient information during these turbulent times have contributed to decision-making by the youth that was not based on correct information. In fact, there is a mythical belief among some caregivers that providing adolescents with information about their bodies and sexuality will result in the early onset of sexual activity. This is not the case. Good research indicates that adolescents with appropriate knowledge are less likely to make decisions that will adversely affect their adolescent years. In other words, they will delay sexual activity, are less likely to fall pregnant, have more confidence and self-esteem, and have better decision-making skills. We cannot afford to have children go unprepared into the world when, today, unsafe sex is very likely to mean death. It is hoped that this book will assist in achieving the objective of providing appropriate information for young people, especially those who do not have caregivers to guide them.

NAIRA KHAN
Director: Child and Law Foundation, Harare

Inequality of the sexes is an injustice prevalent in most societies. So entrenched is it that it is practised and accepted as normal by both men and women.

Two of the commonest excuses for discrimination against women are religion and culture. On the African continent, culture is the most dangerous, and is often used as a weapon to disempower women and, sadly, it is extremely effective. The only way to challenge abusive cultural values is through education. This book provides a first step. Through free discussion and debate the myths about sexual roles and issues can be clarified, and we will be on the road to empowering both sexes.

The basic lessons this book provides are needed by more than just the youth. Parents and grandparents also need to be informed and educated on these matters. Emancipating both men and women will enable us to deal with HIV and the AIDS epidemic much more effectively, and will enhance our ability to preserve our communities and enable them to grow into the future in a positive manner.

Education is the key to liberation, but fair moral values based on equality of human beings need to be promoted by our societies. This book is a promising start. Enjoy reading it and don't let the education be wasted on you.

DR KGOSI LETLAPE
Medical Association of South Africa, Pretoria

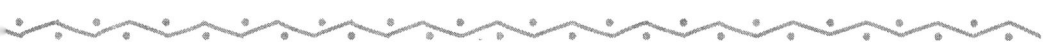

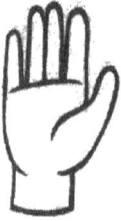

Have you ever wondered ...
whether French kissing is dangerous?
when to break off a relationship?
how to stop your boyfriend from beating you?
what a healthy diet is?
where to go when you find an abandoned baby?
So have we!

We have been created by the publishers, but our questions are real. They are based on actual questions asked by the youth of our region.

This book not only answers our questions, but also provides definitions of many concepts of which we only have a vague understanding. Each word marked with * has a separate entry in the book. Entries are listed alphabetically. Look out for words marked with ♦ because they appear in one of the diagrams on pages 29, 101, 121 and 127 in the book.

On pages 143 and 144 you will find two valuable lists of organisations and agencies with their contact details. These are all specialist help organisations in South Africa and Zimbabwe and can provide you with further advice, and practical assistance in some cases. Please phone them whenever you feel you need to.

At the back you'll also find an index – a list of keywords, with page numbers, so you can look up where the different topics are discussed. Bold numbers indicate the page on which the definition appears and if a word is in bold, in means it has an entry inside the book.

Knowledge is a powerful tool. So enjoy getting informed and empowered!

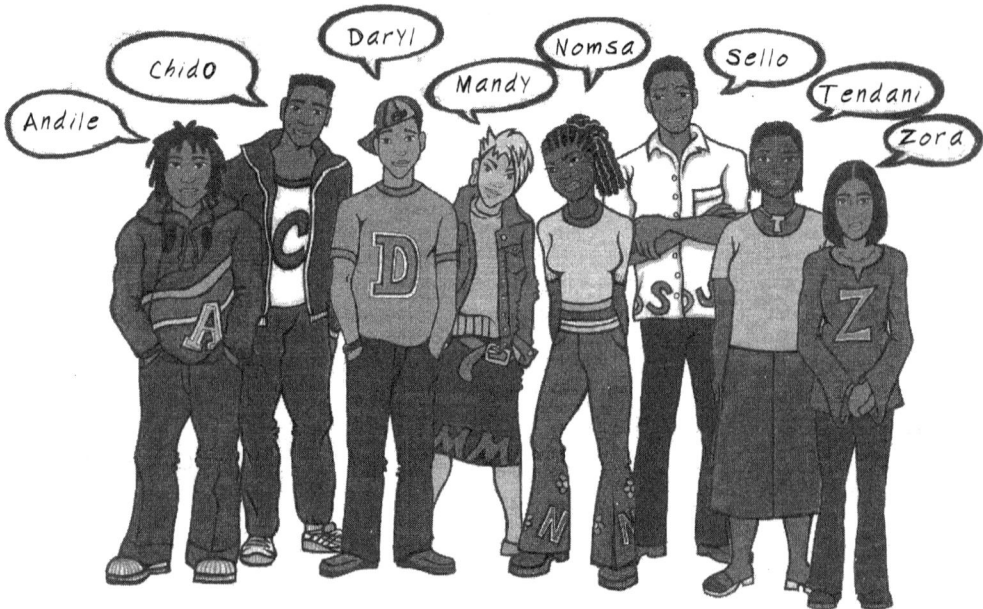

Andile   Chido   Daryl   Mandy   Nomsa   Sello   Tendani   Zora

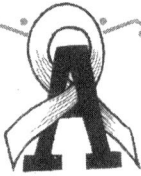

Abortion

Also see **Pregnancy**

An abortion is when the unborn baby is removed from a woman's body to end a pregnancy. Until the unborn baby is 24 weeks old it cannot survive outside of the pregnant mother's body. At this stage the unborn baby is called a foetus or an embryo. After 24 weeks a baby can survive if it is born naturally or by Caesarean section.

What is the difference between abortion and miscarriage?

The words 'abortion' and 'miscarriage' are sometimes used to say the same thing, especially by health workers. However, in common language the word 'miscarriage' is used for when the mother's body rejects the unborn baby because medically something has gone wrong with the pregnancy, whether this is a deliberate or unwanted ending or not. In the case of an 'abortion' the pregnant mother consciously chooses to have her pregnancy ended or terminated, or her doctor advises her to end it for medical reasons.

In Zimbabwe abortion is illegal, but if a woman has tried a self-induced abortion and needs to go to hospital the doctors will sometimes describe it as a miscarriage.

What would make a woman decide to have an abortion?

Living in poverty, being exhausted by having too many children to look after, having no husband or partner to help her feed and educate a child, being seriously ill, or having HIV/AIDS* – these are some of the reasons a woman might wish to end her pregnancy.

An abortion is a serious and traumatic experience, and any woman who undergoes one should receive proper medical care and emotional support. She might have to face religious and social pressure and criticism. However, fear of the attitude of other people should never make her choose a secretive, dangerous abortion. It is very important that an abortion is done by a qualified person, and that the woman tells someone close to her about it so that this person can support her and care for her after the abortion.

But why would someone want to give herself an illegal abortion?

Women who become pregnant, particularly when they have not chosen to become pregnant, often feel very alone. Often they do not have or cannot afford a doctor, sometimes they know their husband or partner would violently disapprove if they were to use contraception, and so they have not been able to exercise control over their own bodies and have become pregnant. Young women or girls who become pregnant often feel so ashamed – they know their parents* will be angry, and very often the man who has made them pregnant abandons them, thus it is desperation which forces them to resort to trying to get rid of the unborn child.

If someone decides to have an abortion, when should it be done?

Abortions should preferably be carried out during the first 14 weeks of pregnancy. If done later, the abortion has to be carried out by inducing labour (actual childbirth*), which is much more traumatic, both physically and emotionally. So if you think that you are pregnant and you have good reasons to consider an abortion, you should get counselling as soon as possible.

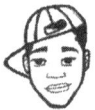

Is abortion legal?

The laws regarding abortion are different in different countries. In some countries abortions are only legal if the woman fell pregnant through rape* or if she is very young. In Zimbabwe abortion is illegal unless giving birth would be a danger to the mother's health, or if the foetus is damaged, or if the pregnancy is a result of rape or incest*. In South Africa it is not against the law to have a pregnancy terminated, on condition that it is done during the first 12 weeks by qualified medical practitioners who can provide proper medical care and psychological support. So-called 'back street' abortions, which are performed without good medical care, are illegal and dangerous. A 'back street' abortion must never be considered, because the pregnant mother can be damaged physically or even die.

In Zimbabwe the penalties against an illegal abortion are severe and women who have given themselves illegal abortions can be imprisoned for up to three years.

What about religion* and abortion?

Different religions have different views on abortion, but most religions do not approve of a woman who chooses to have an abortion. Many religions argue that an abortion amounts to murder, since a potential life is terminated. However, medically, a foetus has a chance of survival only after 24 weeks, so many people do not consider it as a life under 24 weeks.

Many countries in Europe and many states in the USA have legalised abortion in recent decades, allowing that women should have more control over their own bodies. It is recognised that the life of an unwanted child, or a child that a family cannot afford will often not be a very happy one.

Abstinence

Also see Virginity, Marriage

This is when someone chooses not to engage in something, for instance when a person does not drink alcohol* or does not have sexual relations. Such a decision is usually based on moral or religious grounds, or made for health reasons. Many young people choose to abstain from sex until they are married. However, married people sometimes also choose to abstain from sex, e.g. for health reasons or when they don't love each other in a sexual way any more. Abstinence is also a way of avoiding unwanted pregnancies and, of course, HIV/AIDS*.

Is it acceptable to refuse to have sex while you are in a relationship?
Yes, certainly. Sexual intercourse* should make both partners feel good and happy. Therefore it should only happen when both partners agree to it and when they care about each other and are both in the mood for it.

Isn't a bit abnormal not to want to have sex with your boyfriend*?
No, abstinence is a personal choice that all people, young and old, have the right to make. However, if a married person chooses to abstain from sex for a long time without a medical reason, he or she may be unhappy in the relationship. Counselling or talking to a sensible person they trust could help people who feel this way.

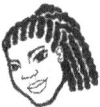

So I have the right not to have sex?
Of course! Nobody should make you have sex against your own wishes. When a man and a woman are married to each other, the law says they have conjugal rights, which means that the couple can reasonably expect their partner to agree to a sexual relationship. For this reason, many people believe that a man has the *right* to have sex with his wife, and that it is her duty to have sex with him. However, the law in both South Africa and Zimbabwe makes it clear that no one has a legal right to force anyone to have sex, not even a husband. If a married man forces his wife to have sex in some societies or countries, including South Africa, he can be charged with rape* and sentenced to prison.

Abuse

Also see **Molesting, Child abuse**

There are different forms of abuse, but all forms of abuse have in common that one person deliberately hurts another human being in the process. Abuse is usually – but not always – physical and means that someone acts violently towards another person, doing him or her harm in the process. The harm can be physical or emotional.

Who is guilty of abuse – only men?

Physical abuse occurs mostly in the form of men hurting women or children, but there are also women who hurt men or children. However, on average men are more aggressive and also stronger, so many more women and children suffer physical abuse and get beaten up than men do.

Does a teacher abuse a schoolchild if he or she spanks the learner?

Hitting a child in order to discipline him or her is called corporal punishment* and in South Africa it is considered abuse. Because it is so easy for people in a position of power, such as teachers, to misuse their position, the physical disciplining of schoolchildren was outlawed in South Africa in 1996. In South Africa only the head of a school may since then give a learner a hiding, and only with the written permission of the parents* and in the presence of another teacher. Teachers who do not comply with these rules can be charged in a court of law. In Zimbabwean schools physical punishment (caning) is allowed only for boys, and must be done by the head of the school in the presence of another staff member, and must be recorded. A parent or guardian can press charges for assault if a child is beaten by a teacher who does not follow the proper procedures.

What about physical abuse towards children?

Yes, many children too suffer physical abuse: friends, family members and even their own parents* sometimes beat them or force them to do hard physical work. Some children are abused sexually – this means that they are used to satisfy an adult's sexual needs, and often they are physically hurt by this because their young bodies are not ready for sexual activity. The emotional damage to the child can also be very severe. And today one of the additional consequences of child rape* is that he or she may contract the HIV virus.

What is emotional abuse*?

There are situations where one person abuses another with words and attitude. A man may, for example, constantly insult his girlfriend* or wife, telling her that she is stupid or ugly, or he can ignore her. Although such a man never physically hurts his partner he nevertheless does great emotional harm to her because his behaviour undermines and destroys her self-esteem and confidence.

But physical abuse also causes emotional damage. This happens because there often is an emotionally close relationship between the abused and the abusive person. Physical hurt is therefore not only an injury to the abused person's body, but also to her feelings and her soul. As a result, the scars from emotional abuse are often more serious and last much longer than the bruises on that person's body.

How can I put an end to abuse?

First of all, find and tell someone you trust and who will believe you and discuss it with him or her. The ideal is a reliable person older than yourself or someone with standing in your community, such as a teacher or a social worker. But anyone you trust is good enough. Ask this person for his or her advice, and then, if there is no alternative course of action that might end the abuse, ask him or her to accompany you to the nearest police station and lay a charge, because the police can protect you.

But remember: not all police are well trained in these matters, and unfortunately it is possible that an unprofessional policeman will believe an abusive man rather than an abused woman or young person. Also remember: before you go to the police, think carefully of what the consequences for your family may be if a police charge is made against your parent or relative or other adult. Make a firm decision then so that nobody can pressurise you to withdraw charges later.

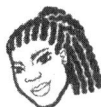

What other outside help is there for abused people?

If you are in an abusive relationship it helps to talk to someone you trust fully. But in addition, and probably before you go to the police, you should get professional help in the form of counselling. A counsellor will talk the situation through with you, and will continue to see you while you deal with the trauma, because often an abused person lacks the confidence or courage to tackle the problem rationally. Empower yourself further by getting educated about your rights and what you really need and want, so that you can take charge of the situation.

What should I do if my boyfriend* beats me but I still love him?

To be physically abused by another human being is never, under any circumstances, acceptable. The short answer is: leave him. Otherwise you might even reach a point where you see the abuse as a sign of affection and say to yourself: 'My boyfriend has taken notice of me, he beats me! He minded what I did, so he cares, that's why he beats me!'

If you find yourself in an abusive relationship it is unlikely that the abuser will change his ways, even though he might promise to do so. Experiences of abusive relationships show that the abuse will most likely get worse, so the sooner you break up with your boyfriend (or husband) the better.

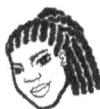

How can I prevent being beaten by my boyfriend?

It is very important to remember that it is not your fault if you have an abusive boyfriend.

Nobody is perfect, but we all have the right to our own opinions and ideas and the way we are. If you can't discuss your differences with your boyfriend without him becoming violent then you should leave him, or seek counselling, or do both.

Why does my boyfriend beat me?

Even though you, like many other victims of abuse, may blame yourself and believe that you have said or done something 'wrong' that angered your boyfriend and caused him to beat you, this is never the real reason. Even if you have worn an outfit he hates, or said something he resents, he still does not have any right to beat you. In some social groups or societies it is not considered abnormal for husbands to beat wives, but the laws of most countries do not accept this macho* attitude. People who are physically violent are often very damaged themselves – they may have been beaten as children, or they are so deeply insecure in themselves that they cannot tolerate any kind of difference. It is a known fact that many abusers have been abused themselves, so they abuse other people in turn. Therefore, unless counselling is sought, this vicious cycle will continue.

What causes domestic violence?

There are so many possible reasons for domestic violence: for instance the man and woman may not love each other any more, but neither of them can make the decision to leave, because they are still emotionally or economically dependent on one another. Other reasons may be: alcohol* abuse; one of the partners suffering from a sense of inferiority or experiencing a low morale in the workplace; a shortage of money, sexual frustration, or because they believe their partner is being unfaithful. All these factors may contribute to domestic violence. So the best advice for families experiencing domestic violence is to seek professional advice, counselling and support.

It is often very difficult to convince victims of domestic violence to seek outside help, because they are usually afraid, feel helpless and have lost hope, so they prefer to suffer in silence. But the only way to break the cycle of violence is to find the courage to speak to a respected relative or to contact one of the help organisations. Most of these organisations, such as Life Line or Connect, can be contacted 24 hours a day, and the people working there are sympathetic and helpful.

Addiction

Also see Alcohol, Drugs, Smoking

Addiction is when a person's body cannot function properly without a certain substance, such as drugs*, tobacco (nicotine) or alcohol*. An addicted person has introduced the substance so regularly into his or her body that it has become dependent on the substance. Once someone has become dependent on or addicted to something, his or her mind and body cannot operate well without that substance.

Adoption

When a person or a couple adopt a child they take over the legal responsibility of looking after and caring for all the legal, social, educational and moral needs of a child who is not theirs by birth.

How does a child get adopted?
Usually children become available for adoption because at birth, their parents* are not able to care for them. An individual or a couple who wish to adopt a child have to follow certain legal procedures. Rules of adoption vary from country to country, but generally the family life and financial situation of prospective adoptive parents are considered, as well as their age and ability to care for a child. Sometimes relatives of an orphaned child who lost both parents adopt the child, but more often it is done by other people who are unable to have children of their own. A child can be adopted from birth right up to the legal age of majority, which is 18 years.

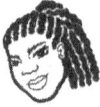

What do adoption agencies do?

They are organisations that specialise in putting together potential parents – carefully investigating their suitability as prospective parents – and children who do not have parents to care for them. They handle all the legal aspects of adoption and some operate across different countries and even continents. In Zimbabwe, however, only the Department of Social Welfare is legally permitted to arrange adoptions.

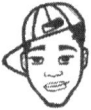

Does the adopted child ever get to know her or his birth parents?

It was previously felt that adopted children should never know their biological parents. However, a recent approach in some countries is that an adopted child has a right to this information. Sometimes birth parents may be difficult to trace, and might not want to meet a child they have given up for adoption. So the adopted child who wants to find his birth parents should be prepared for the possibility of disappointment or rejection, but in many cases the birth parents are happy that their child cared enough to look for them.

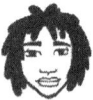

What are the rights of the birth father?

If the father and mother of a child are married to each other and the mother wants to give the child up for adoption the father has to give his consent, unless he has deserted the child or failed to look after it without any good reason. Only the mother's consent is needed if she is unmarried and the father has failed to contribute to maintaining the child, or denies that he is the father of the child. The same applies to a child born as a result of rape* or incest*.

How does taboo* impact on abortion*?

In some African countries, people are very reluctant to adopt children if they do not know a child, or who his or her ancestors are. They fear that if the child becomes ill they will not know which spirits to appease. As an alternative, many families in Africa arrange to care for, or 'adopt', the children of a sister or brother, especially if they cannot have their own.

Adultery

Adultery is committed when a person has sexual intercourse* with someone else's legally married husband or wife.

Can adultery be punished?

Adultery is usually considered a civil offence, which means that the husband or wife whose partner committed adultery can sue the person who became sexually involved with their partner. However, in some circumstances adultery is considered a crime, for example, according to fundamentalist Muslim law, it is a crime and the guilty party may be punished with imprisonment or even death.

Most religions* have firm views on adultery and consider it a sin, but unless the laws of a religion are also the laws of a state, adultery is not an offence punishable by law.

But what about having two wives?

In some religions, such as Islam and some traditional African beliefs, it is perfectly acceptable for a man to have more than one wife.

In Western societies that follow Christian guidelines, marriage* is usually monogamous, which means it is a partnership between only two people. But the growing tendency towards divorce* means that a man or a woman can be married more than once in the course of their life. Most Protestant Christian churches accept this practice, but the Catholic church does not recognise divorce, even if the partners no longer live together. This means that if a divorced Catholic remarries, he or she does it against the rules of their church. However, in special circumstances, a marriage which has not been consummated may be annulled.

AIDS see HIV/AIDS

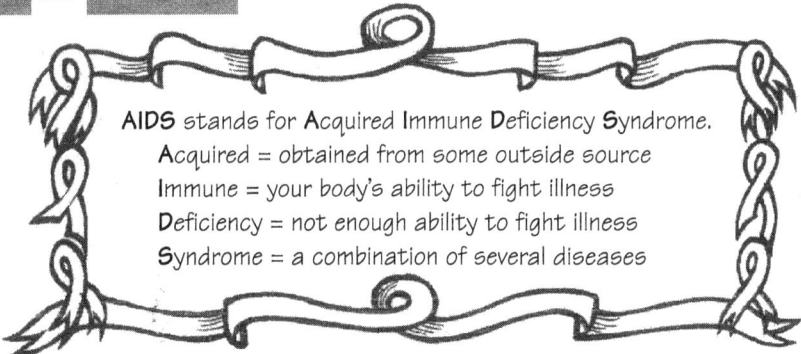

AIDS stands for Acquired Immune Deficiency Syndrome.
Acquired = obtained from some outside source
Immune = your body's ability to fight illness
Deficiency = not enough ability to fight illness
Syndrome = a combination of several diseases

Alcohol

Alcohol is a substance found in certain drinks, such as wine, beer, brandy, whisky, rum and so forth. Alcohol alters your brain functions and influences people to behave differently from when they are sober: some people become silly, or sleepy, others aggressive. When people become dependent on alcohol, they have become addicted to it.

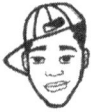

How does alcohol affect people?

'Having a drink' and 'drinking' are two different things. When people drink alcohol in moderate quantities while having a good conversation and being social, it can make them relaxed and enjoy themselves. However, when people consume too much alcohol it usually causes them to be uninhibited, or rude, or abusive, or violent, or silly, or downright boring, or they fall asleep – or all of these! Some people also become irresponsible because they cannot think straight when they have had too much to drink. They also become uncoordinated and cannot walk straight or talk properly. This is why companies warn people not to operate machinery when they have been drinking.

Also, too much drinking results in an unpleasant hangover*!

What about drinking and driving?

This is a serious matter! Drunkenness is a major cause of car accidents, and can cause damage to or the death of innocent people. For this reason it is an offence against the law to drive under the influence of liquor. If one is caught for drunken driving by the police you will receive a fine or will be punished in another way, depending on the laws of the country and on whether you have caused an accident. Your driver's licence can be endorsed or taken away and you might even receive a jail sentence if you have caused someone's death.

What are 'moderate quantities' and what is 'too much' when you drink?

Some people can hold their alcohol well; others need to be much more careful. Knowing your limits is very important.

In Zimbabwe if your alcohol content is more than 0.08 g per 100 ml of blood you can be prosecuted. In South Africa you may not drive if you have more than 0.05 g of alcohol per 100 ml of blood in your body. The average guidelines for staying within these limits are not to exceed 2 glasses of wine, 2 cans of beer or 2 tots of hard liquor if you weigh about 70 kg. The lower your body weight, the faster you will reach the legal limit, so the less you weigh the less you should drink! If you are 18 years or older and you stick to these quantities you will be within the limits of the law – and should also not suffer from a hangover* the next day!

Just remember that spirits such as vodka or gin are often mixed with something sweet, so you do not taste the alcohol and do not realise that you might be drinking far more than you should.

At what age is it acceptable to start drinking?

In many societies young people start to drink alcohol too early when they don't really want to and can't manage it, but they do it because of peer pressure*. In other words someone feels obliged to start drinking alcohol because all their friends are drinking, even though they might not like the sensation, get drunk, feel sick and develop hangovers.

Eighteen is the age at which one legally becomes an adult and is allowed to drink in most southern African countries.

People who do not drink alcohol out of moral or religious conviction say that children should never be given alcohol to drink. Other adults reason that it is not a bad idea to expose children in their teens to small amounts of wine or beer because in this way they get used to drinking in moderation and will not think of drinking as a 'thrilling forbidden fruit'.

Medically speaking, most people who start drinking small amounts of alcohol around the age of 16 do not suffer great harm. But serious problems arise when someone hangs around with others who think it is cool to drink heavily and, for example, boast about how many beers they can down in one hour. This can lead to you getting into the habit of drinking heavily and becoming addicted to alcohol because of peer pressure. A pregnant woman can damage her unborn baby if she drinks more than a very small amount of alcohol.

The important thing to remember is that there is no age at which you *have* to start drinking. It is not necessary at all to drink if you do not want to or don't feel like it or if it is against your principles.

Why does alcohol make people lose control?

Alcohol takes away your inhibitions. This means that you may say and do things that you would feel too shy to do or say if you were sober. So even though a drink can relax you, too much alcohol may cause you to lose control of yourself and do things that you later regret, or cannot even remember properly.

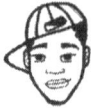

Does alcohol make people feel sexy?

Some, but not all, people experience erotic feelings and become sexually aroused when they have consumed alcohol. However, this is because alcohol makes people less shy and not because alcohol is an aphrodisiac*. Under the influence of alcohol they lose the inhibitions which normally make them repress their sexual feelings.

How does alcohol affect sexual performance?

Alcohol may increase sexual desire by reducing inhibitions, but it also reduces sexual performance because it can make you clumsy or drowsy. And it impairs judgement. People who have had too much to drink are far less likely to take the precaution of using a condom* to prevent the transmission of HIV/AIDS* and other sexually transmitted infections (STIs)*. So by not bothering to wear a condom they are putting their lives and the lives of their partners in danger.

What is an alcoholic?

There is a difference between someone who is an alcoholic and someone who is a heavy drinker. An alcoholic is dependent on alcohol and cannot live without it. It is not easy to define the condition scientifically, because it relates to the individual ways in which people's bodies and minds behave. However, there are some common tell-tale signs of alcoholism. These include when someone:
- drinks alone, or is very secretive about drinking,
- drinks large amounts of alcohol in a short space of time (binge drinking),
- steals money to buy liquor,
- starts to drink early in the morning,
- shakes when he or she is sober,
- drinks undiluted sugar-cane spirits and even methylated spirits (both of which are very dangerous, as they can make you blind),
- suffers from severe mood swings,
- needs another alcoholic drink to get rid of a hangover*,
- boasts about his or her drinking habits,
- experiences a loss of memory and
- has a body odour* of stale alcohol.

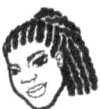

Is heavy drinking a threat to my health?

Yes. Usually, it takes several years of heavy drinking for someone to develop a serious addiction and the health problems that follow, but in some cases it can take as little as one year. Besides alcoholism affecting one's memory and judgement it can cause mood swings and even severe malnutrition, when alcoholics consume only drink and don't bother to eat properly. Alchohol contains a lot of sugar, so drinking too much alcohol can lead to being overweight (obesity*). Finally, excessive long-term drinking and alcoholism affect your health: your liver, heart and nervous system will not work effectively any more. In addition alcoholics suffer from shaking and tremors.

How can I help an alcoholic?

Don't nag someone who drinks, but don't support the person's drinking habit either. If you live with the person, do not keep alcohol in the house. If it is a friend, try to meet in places where there is no alcohol. Do not drink alcohol in the presence of the person.

Alcoholics are often very difficult to live with because of their unpredictable emotional behaviour, their inability to hold onto a job, their secretiveness and the amount of money they spend on alcohol. But when they are sober, heavy drinkers can be very pleasant; it is only when they are intoxicated that their moods are difficult to cope with.

It can be heartbreaking to see someone that you love or like very much ruining their lives with alcohol abuse. However, an alcoholic needs emotional support. Alcoholics are often unhappy people who drink to try and forget about the pain they are feeling.

There is not much point in telling an alcoholic he or she has a problem if they do not want to face the fact. So before you can really help a person with a drinking problem, that person has to admit to him- or herself that they have such a problem. Once an alcoholic person has taken this step you can provide important support, such as going to Alcoholics Anonymous (AA)* meetings with them, not drinking alcohol in their presence and encouraging them to remain sober.

Alcoholics Anonymous (AA)

It is a self-help organisation to support people who recognise that they have a drinking problem. The AA holds regular support meetings where members can share their problems. It also offers a 'friend' system whereby a member can telephone someone if he or she feels they are in danger of drinking alcohol again. The AA works on the basis that once you are an alcoholic you are always an alcoholic and can never risk taking a drink again. The only solution is to abstain from drinking altogether. The AA has a sister organisation called Alanon, which provides support for the families of alcoholics.

Anal sex

Also see **Sodomy**

Anal sex is sexual intercourse* during which one person enters the other person's body through the rectum* or anus*. It is a fairly common practice between homosexual* lovers, but also occurs between men and women.

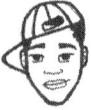

Is anal sex enjoyable?

Some people think so and prefer to have sex in this way, others find it painful. Anyone brought up to believe it is 'unnatural' and wrong, and a 'sin', might find it hard to accept this practice. One important thing should be remembered however: because the tissue in the anus is fragile, the skin tears easily. It is therefore all the more important to use a condom* during anal sex, because the slightest wound can lead to a sexually transmitted infection* or virus, should your partner be HIV*-positive.

Anorexia

This is an extreme and potentially fatal medical condition. It arises when someone, usually a young woman, deprives her body of food in order to lose weight, or forces herself to vomit any food she may have eaten. The habit of depriving the body of food becomes so damaging that the person eventually cannot eat at all, and the body rejects any food taken in. If not identified and treated early, an anorexic person can die of starvation.

Girls who become anorexic often do so as a result of dieting. They feel they are 'too fat', although this is usually a very subjective judgement and one that reveals their own deep insecurities. Once they begin to diet* they find themselves unable to stop.

Today we live in a world that is strongly influenced by advertising, which often uses women's bodies to sell products, and they will use models who are often very slim. So thinness subconsciously becomes equated with beauty and success.

However, remember that not everyone who is very thin has anorexia. Some people are naturally thin, and do not eat much.

My girlfriend* has stopped eating – what can I do?

Often there is very little that friends or family can do once a young woman becomes obsessive about wanting to lose weight. Give her as much support and reassurance as you can, and advise her to see a doctor and a counsellor or therapist. Most girls who are unhappy about their weight are unhappy about themselves and judge themselves very harshly in comparison to other people.

Aphrodisiac

These are potions that a man (and sometimes a woman) will eat or drink believing they will improve their sex drive. Aphrodisiacs range from herbs to rhino-horn powder. Most aphrodisiacs do nothing physically and people's sexual performance seems better only because they believe subconsciously that the potion is taking effect.

Recently men who suffer from impotence[*] (the inability to have an erection or to keep an erection long enough to have sexual intercourse) have started to use Viagra[*], a medication which causes more blood to flow to the penis[*]. However, Viagra is not an ordinary aphrodisiac because it does not alter people's sex drive as such – it is a help only to men with a physical problem.

Attraction

There are many different kinds of attraction: emotional, sexual, mental, etc. Attraction is something in another person that you either like, appreciate or find interesting and which draws you to that person. An initial attraction is often based on physical beauty or charm, but other factors such as personality, common interests and shared activities and values determine whether the attraction will last. Superficial sexual attraction, based only on a person's physical appearance and not supported by shared beliefs and interests and a real liking, usually doesn't last very long. Mutual attraction (when both people are attracted to each other) is often immediate, but it can form the basis for a more permanent relationship.

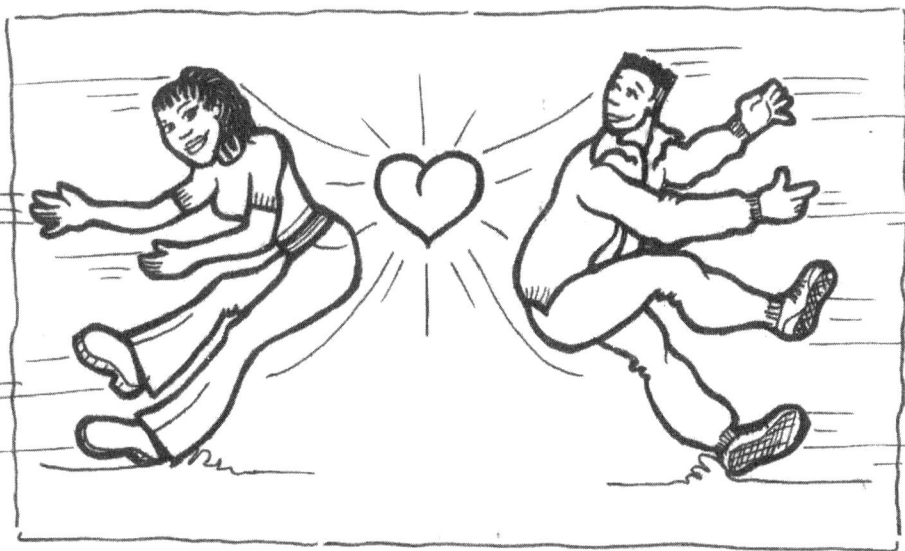

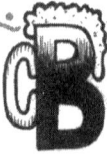

Baby dumping

Baby dumping is when a mother abandons her baby by leaving it somewhere, usually in the hope that the baby will be found and cared for.

Why would a woman want to dump her baby?

When a young woman becomes pregnant she often is poor, alone (both parents* may have died) or she has dropped out of school, and her future looks bleak. Often she has met a young man who flatters her and who she believes wants to marry her. Instead, he takes advantage of her, and then dumps her. Frequently the pregnant girl is too scared to tell her mother or father that she is pregnant, and feels alone and lost and does not know what to do without anyone to support her. Often she hides her pregnancy* from everyone, cannot afford to go to the clinic, has the baby in secret, and then leaves it somewhere hoping that someone will find it and look after it.

If the baby is found it is the young mother who is prosecuted, not the boy who made her pregnant in the first place. Many people believe that had the girl received the right kind of advice and emotional support she would never have dumped the baby, which was an act of desperation.

In Zimbabwe and South Africa homes and shelters have been founded for pregnant girls who have been abandoned by their boyfriends or thrown out of their families.

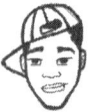

How does the law react to a mother who has dumped her baby?

Although society has become more aware that such women are more to be pitied than blamed, the law penalises baby-dumpers severely. A mother who has abandoned her baby has committed an offence and can be charged and sentenced to a fine or a term in prison. If the child dies the parent who has abandoned the baby might be charged with murder.

By failing to look after a child and putting its life or health in danger a parent may lose the right to take care of the child in future. A court may rule that the baby be taken away from the mother who has dumped it and be placed in a foster home or given up for adoption*.

The South African Child Care Act states that any parent who abandons a child shall be guilty of an offence. It is thus considered a crime when a person unlawfully and intentionally exposes and abandons an infant in a place or in circumstances where the child could possibly suffer death from exposure. If a parent abandons the child with the intent to kill it, that person can be found guilty of murder. Abandonment (dumping) which results in the accidental death of a child can result in a charge of culpable homicide (unintentional manslaughter). To abandon a dead child is also an offence in South Africa.

In Zimbabwe it is an offence to wilfully abandon a baby – 'baby dumping' – but greater understanding of the desperation of the mothers has given rise to more lenient sentences, such as community service.

What should I do if I find an abandoned baby?

Firstly, it is important that you keep it warm and immediately get help, then to take it to the nearest police station or hospital or clinic or, if you are concerned about harming the baby, phone the police or hospital and ask them for assistance and advice. If you can't phone, get the help of an adult whom you know and trust. If you know where the nearest welfare organisation is that deals with child adoption*, you could also approach them for assistance. The main thing is to report that you have found an abandoned baby and to get outside professional help quickly. You should not believe or hope that you or your family could keep the baby and care for it.

Can women who feel they can't keep their baby find help somewhere?

A woman who feels that she can't take responsibility for her baby can approach the nearest welfare or church organisation, where someone will guide and assist her. They will help her make the best decision for her self and her baby. Childline* will also assist in such cases.

Bad breath

Bad breath is when a person's breath smells unpleasant. It is called 'halitosis' in medical terms. It can have various causes: not cleaning your teeth properly, bad teeth, constipation or poor digestion.

My boyfriend* has bad breath. What can I do about it?

First try to find out what is causing the problem. Then try to raise it with him.

You have to treat this sensitively, because you might offend your boyfriend. You could try making a joke about it, for example by saying, 'So-and-so has such bad breath, he should really try to eat more roughage.'

If your boyfriend does not take the hint you will have to talk to him about it openly.

Being faithful see Faithfulness

Birth control

Also see Contraception, Family planning

Birth control is what a couple does when they avoid having unwanted babies. They can do this by not having sexual intercourse* (abstinence*) or by using one of the various methods of contraception.

Body odour (BO)

When someone smells unpleasant, usually like stale sweat, it is called body odour.

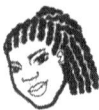

One of my classmates always smells of sweat. Should I tell him?
You could try to raise it with him and suggest that he washes more regularly and perhaps uses deodorant. However, you have to treat it sensitively, because you might offend him. You could try making a joke about it, for example by saying, 'So-and-so smells terrible, he should really use deodorant.' If your classmate does not take the hint you will have to talk to him about it openly.

Boyfriend

Also see Faithfulness, Commitment, Dating

A boyfriend can be described as a girl's or woman's usual or favourite companion.

When can I call someone my boyfriend?
When there is a warm feeling of love* and affection and loyalty between a boy and a girl, and neither of them have intimate physical contact with any other boy or girl, the relationship is that of a boyfriend and girlfriend*. A boyfriend is a man with whom you can share your worries, joys and fears. It is usually a good thing if your parents* know your boyfriend, as this may help to ensure that he won't take advantage of you or force you to do anything you are not ready for, like getting involved in a sexual relationship.

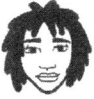

May a girl tell her boyfriend what she wants?

Traditionally, it was frowned upon for girls to express their likes and dislikes, or even their opinions. Girls were expected to be submissive and to wait for the boy to take the lead. Some people, because of particular religious or cultural beliefs, still feel that this ought to be the way to do things, but today girls should feel confident, and where necessary even insist, to tell her boyfriend what she wants.

May I tell my boyfriend that he must change his attitude?

Yes, certainly, although it is always advisable to do it in a polite way. If your boyfriend is very macho*, he might get angry and walk out on you. If he does that you need to ask yourself: Do I really want to be with some-body who has this attitude and behaves in this way? If the answer is 'No' then you should not feel bad if he 'dumps' you.

Finding out who you really are and what is important to you is part of growing up. Finding out if your boyfriend will allow you to be the person you feel you are, and how he behaves towards you, is a valuable and continuous process. Only by being honest with him will you get to know him, and if you might want to marry or live with him one day.

In an equal society girls need to understand their rights and learn to assert themselves. This does not mean that they need to be aggressive and not respect their boyfriends' feelings and opinions or try to impose their will on them. On the other hand, their boyfriends must equally respect their girlfriends' wishes and ideas. This does not always happen, as many men still do not really accept that girls have rights. Often they want to control their girlfriends as if they were their possessions.

Is it OK to have sex with my boyfriend?

Yes, on condition that you feel comfortable with your decision and under-stand the implications. If you have sex with him only because you fear that if you say 'no' he will break off the relationship and 'dump' you, or because you fear that your friends will make fun of you and call you 'old-fashioned' or 'frigid' (see frigidity*), you should perhaps think again.

Unless there is mutual love* and mutual respect*, having sex is not even pleasurable. If your partner demands that you have sex with him against your wishes or your principles, it probably means that he doesn't respect you and is a selfish person who is concerned only with his own needs and wishes.

It is important to discuss your feelings about sex with him. If you feel that you are not ready to become sexually active your boyfriend should be able to respect and accept this.

On the other hand, if you have decided to become sexually involved with him, you must remember that there are some serious responsibilities: you need to have knowledge of contraception* to avoid pregnancy*, as well know how to protect yourself against sexually transmitted infections (STIs)* and/or HIV/AIDS*.

How do I prevent my friends from seducing my boyfriend?

One can't really control what other people do. If a friend seduces your boyfriend then she is not a true friend, because she does not care about your feelings. Also, if this happens your boyfriend is not a very loyal or trustworthy person, and you are better off without him. Choose your friends and boyfriend very carefully. It always hurts when someone betrays you, but it does happen. It is part of life. In the end it shows us whom we can trust and whom not.

What should I do if my boyfriend tells me that he no longer loves me?

First of all, don't think that there is anything wrong with you! Remember that he is not 'the only fish in the river' and that there are other nice men around. If he doesn't love you, you are in any case better off without him. Give yourself a few treats: buy a new lipstick, change your hairstyle, go dancing with a friend. Keep yourself busy by doing something new, like developing a new hobby – reading or singing in the school or church choir, or doing sport. Tell yourself that your happiness does not depend on him and that you can have fun without him. Don't try to get him back at all costs!

Bride-price see Lobola

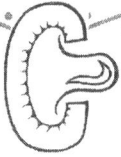

Caesarean section

A Caesarean section is a surgical operation which is performed to deliver a baby when natural childbirth* is impossible. This is usually done when the unborn baby is at risk or showing signs of distress, or if the mother's birth canal* is too narrow. In such cases the doctor cuts through the mother's skin and through the wall of her womb in order to reach the baby inside her. However, as prenatal care has improved, and as there are so many ways of checking on the health of the unborn baby and the mother during pregnancy*, fewer Caesareans are performed these days.

However, Caesarean births are common practice when the mother is HIV-positive because they reduce the risk of the baby becoming infected during childbirth.

Child abuse

Child abuse is when physical or emotional harm is caused to a child. This includes depriving a child of food, water or warmth; locking a child up in a room for long periods of time; denying a child education*; forcing a child to do hard physical work; sending a child to beg in the streets, or exposing a child to prostitution* or drugs*.

Sexually molesting* and raping children are two of the most serious forms of child abuse. The abuse can take the form of simply touching parts of the child's body and touching the child in such a way that makes the child feel uncomfortable. Sexual abuse of children can also mean persuading or forcing them to perform sexual acts such as oral sex* and sexual intercourse*.

Who abuses children sexually?
A boy can be sexually abused by a grown man or grown woman; likewise a girl can be abused by an adult of either gender*. Children of any age – even babies of a few months – can be the victims of abuse. Adults who are sexually attracted to children are called paedophiles*. Two of the worst types of abuse are when children are forced into the sex trade as sex workers* or when they are forced to act in pornographic* films.

Unfortunately today some men infected with the HIV* virus are led to believe that if they have sex with a virgin – which is often interpreted as short-hand for 'child' – they will be cured. This has led to a rise in the incidence of child rape*. The man is not, of course, cured; the child suffers terrible emotional and physical hurt, and may well acquire the HIV virus.

A girl in our class was abused by her uncle – does this often happen?
Unfortunately most people who molest children are known to the child, and may well be a member of the family. They are people who otherwise live very ordinary lives, often with wives, children and friends of their own. We often think that a person who abuses a child must be insane, some kind of ogre or monster, but the reverse is true. In fact, it is only a minority of children who are abused by strangers.

Where can a sexually abused child go for help?
Very often an abused child does not tell anyone what is happening, because the adult who abuses the child is someone that the child knows well and whom the child has trusted. And sometimes when an abused child does try to tell her or his parents* the parents find it difficult to believe the child because the abuser is often a friend of the family, or an uncle or an aunt, or even one of the parents. It is, however, very important for children to tell someone about the abuse, however hard it is to talk about it. The obvious person would be a parent, but if it is not possible to talk to a parent they can perhaps talk to an aunt or a teacher. Childline*, a special free phone-in and write-in service for children, specifically provides support and assistance to children.

What happens if a sexually abused child keeps quiet?
It is very important for any child who is being abused to tell someone about it or ask for help. An abused person can never just forget about the experience. On the contrary: an abused person nearly always takes a great amount of hidden anger and a misplaced sense of guilt into adulthood, which can makes it difficult for her or him to form loving relationships later.

Also, if the paedophile* is not stopped she or he will continue to abuse children.

What should I do if I know of a little girl who is being abused?
If the child is too scared to tell anyone else, make her understand that she can talk to you and that you will believe what she tells you. If her parents are not sympathetic, or if they are somehow involved, you might want to make it clear that you will not tell them about it. Remember that the little girl may be frightened to talk because the abusing adult might have told her that if she tells anybody something dreadful will happen. In such a case

you need to reassure her that this will not happen. Once she has taken you into her confidence you need to seek professional help, for example through Childline* or a social worker, your local doctor or a nurse. Childline* can be telephoned at any time, day or night.

Do not try to confront the abuser: leave that to the professionals and the police!

In Zimbabwe people still practise ngozi; isn't this a form of child abuse?
The practice of giving a girl to the family of a man who has been murdered by a member of the culprit's family is illegal in Zimbabwe, though many people still practise this traditional custom. If a girl feels herself threatened by such a situation she should get in touch with Childline* or report it to a trusted teacher, who will take up the matter with the police.

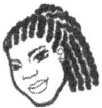

Child betrothal also happens in Zimbabwe; is this not also a form of abuse?
Some traditionalists and members of certain religious sects still betroth young girls to men much older than themselves, who are often already married with families. Should you know of anyone in this situation who does not want to get married you should contact Childline* or a trusted teacher.

Childbirth

Also see *Pregnancy*

Childbirth (labour) usually happens spontaneously about 280 days (nine months) after the baby was conceived. (A first baby may take a little longer before it is ready to be born.) Childbirth is a process that starts when the muscular wall of the uterus* begins to contract. In the beginning the contractions are far apart, but the closer it gets to the baby being born the more regular they become. Next the muscles of the cervix* (the neck of the womb) relax. Then the mother's water – the amniotic sac surrounding and protecting the baby – breaks and the contractions of the uterus

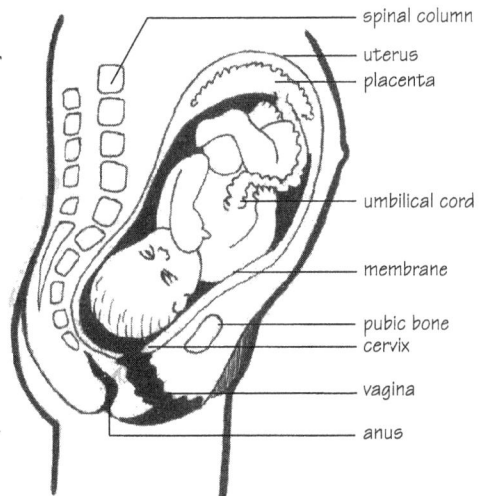

- spinal column
- uterus
- placenta
- umbilical cord
- membrane
- pubic bone
- cervix
- vagina
- anus

muscles push the baby into the cervix, head first, and then out through the vagina*. The umbilical cord* that connects the baby to the mother's womb* must now be cut, and the baby lifted up and lightly smacked so that it can cry to open its lungs to the air outside the mother's body. Finally, the afterbirth – the placenta* and membranes in the womb which have fed and protected the baby during pregnancy – is delivered.

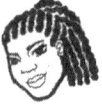

What is the ideal age to have a child?

Some cultures think it is fine for teenage girls to have babies, others think a woman should at least be in her twenties. Biologically it is best for a woman to have a child when she is younger and fitter, between 18 and 24 years. If the mother is over 36 years old the chances of a first child being born with a defect are greater. Emotionally, however, a mother needs to be mature enough to handle the responsibility of raising a child. The trend in Africa is towards women having children once they have reached the age of majority, 18, and are married. Generally speaking, a woman in her twenties is more mature than a teenager, and it is always best to postpone having children until you feel you can support them financially and emotionally.

What about much older women having children?

Medical science has developed so much in recent times that it is now possible for a woman to have a child even in her sixties. This is because of artificial fertilisation, a process by which a cell from a fertile woman is fertilised outside of the body and then the fertilised egg is returned to the body of the woman who will bear the child. Some people argue that this is immoral because such a practice interferes with nature, which determines that women generally become infertile after 55, because they stop menstruating* and producing fertile cells. Another argument against having children at a very mature age is that older parents* are more likely to die before the child has grown up.

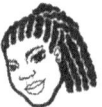

Is having a child dangerous? What can go wrong?

Having a baby is a perfectly normal activity. Very little should go wrong if the mother is healthy and has attended a prenatal clinic regularly, and if she has done exercises to strengthen her stomach muscles – especially if she has her baby delivered in a hospital or clinic, or at home with a midwife in attendance.

However, there are a number of problems that may arise, one of the commonest being a 'breech birth', where the unborn child is positioned the wrong way round, with the feet instead of the head pointing downwards.

When this is the case a doctor will often advise a Caesarean section[*] to make sure that the baby is delivered safely.

Another complication is if labour takes longer than eight to 12 hours, because it can tire out the mother so much that she does not have enough energy to complete the whole process of childbirth.

Also, if the mother is ill, or if she gives birth without the assistance of a qualified person, complications such as heavy bleeding or *obstructed labour* (when the baby turns horizontal and can't move down the birth canal) can arise.

And, of course, teenage mothers, whose bodies and wombs are not fully developed, may have difficulty and experience severe pain when giving birth because their birth passage is too narrow. When this happens both the child and the mother will tire more easily and a Caesarean section might become necessary.

When the baby is born prematurely (before the pregnancy has run the full course of 280 days or nine months) many complications can occur. Then the baby has to be kept in a hospital in special care.

Childline

Childline is a South African organisation that helps children and young people who have been victims of abuse[*]. Callers who dial the number 08000 55555 will receive advice or support from a trained counsellor. The number is toll-free, which means it is free. The line is open 24 hours a day. The Childline counsellor will help an abused child or young person to talk about what has happened to him or her, and will suggest what can be done to stop it from happening. In Gauteng Childline also offers treatment centres and safe houses. In Zimbabwe the number to call from anywhere in the country is 961; or you can call Harare 701111/2.

Cigarettes (tobacco) see Smoking

Co-habitation

Co-habitation, also called 'living together', is when a couple live together without being legally married. In modern Western societies this is becoming more common as men and women become more cautious about getting married and as society becomes more accepting of this form of partnership. However, co-habitation is also a traditional practice in societies where a man is entitled to have more than one customary-law wife. This is called polygamy[*].

In Zimbabwe if a couple do not register their partnership through a legal marriage*, or perform the necessary customary-law requirements, should the relationship fall apart neither party has any defined legal rights. Usually the girl loses out, as generally property is registered in the man's name.

Does a couple who co-habit have the same rights as married people?

Generally, if a couple live together without having drawn up any form of marriage contract, their relationship does not have any legal status. If they have children the children will be under the guardianship of the mother, but the father will be required to pay maintenance.

Generally, in terms of the tax law a married couple have advantages over two single working people who are taxed separately.

In some countries people who have lived together for a considerable time are considered to have the same legal status as a married couple. This does not apply in Zimbabwe. In South Africa people who co-habit can argue a case for receiving the same rights and benefits as a married couple, e.g. medical aid, but it is not an automatic right.

My aunt and uncle lived together for a long time before they got married. No one thought it was wrong. Was it?

No, of course not. In customary law if a man and woman get married and the bride price* is paid after they have had children, the father of the 'bride' will ask for damages in addition to the lobola* payment. This is often agreed affectionately and without any sense of 'damage' as there would be if his daughter had been raped.

What is a mapoto wife?

Sometimes migrant workers find themselves a temporary wife – a 'mapoto wife' – because they are working and living in the mining towns, far away from home. Men in prison sometimes make similar arrangements with men, because there are no women in prison. In Zimbabwe, the term 'kapoto' describes a man who is 'used as a wife' in prison. The kapotos in prison tend to be younger, smaller men. They may be weaker men who are very unwilling to take on this role, but are forced into it.

Mapoto wives may look after a man for many years but they have no rights should he die.

Commitment

Being committed to someone or to a relationship means that you are prepared to try your best to resolve problems or differences because you have made a promise to yourself and the other person about the relationship. Commitment to a relationship is the basis for faithfulness*.

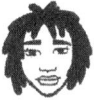

Is commitment necessary in a relationship?

If you want a relationship between you and a girl to last, or for it to have emotional depth, you must keep to the promises you and she have made to each other and remain loyal. Commitment to a girlfriend* is a sign of how seriously you regard your relationship with her.

Compatibility

This is when people get along very well, usually because they share the same values and attitudes, as well as interests and hobbies, such as reading, taking part in sport or watching TV. Two people with the same principles, from the same social background or culture, with similar education* and who belong to the same religion* or belief system also tend to be more compatible than if they differed completely in all these respects. However, there are many examples of couples who are happy together even though they are very different from each other. In such cases people say: 'opposites attract'. Nobody knows exactly what makes people compatible.

Is it possible to live with and love someone of a different religion?

It is strange, but often a couple finds it easier to live with major differences – e.g. one person being a Christian and the other a Hindu, or one person being a church-goer and the other not – than for them to accept small differences. People might accept religious difference but argue about small matters, such as tidiness, taste in clothing, even table manners*.

So it is better to get to know someone very well before you marry him or her. It is no good, for example, finding out too late that you want one child and your partner is planning to have four! If you are dating* someone and are thinking of getting married or living with that person permanently, it is important to discuss big as well as small issues.

Whether you can be happy with someone who does not belong to the same religion as you would depend on whether there is true mutual respect* in your relationship and an appreciation of each other's differences.

Condom

Also see **Contraception, Family planning**

A condom is a contraceptive that covers the penis* and is used by men to protect them from infections and from conceiving unwanted children. It comes in the form of a rolled-up flexible sheath made out of a fine but strong material, such as latex. To be effective a man must put the condom on his penis before he enters a woman's body and has sex with her. It must be kept on throughout sexual intercourse*.

Why do men use condoms?

A condom is a device used for contraception. It protects men from making unwanted babies because the semen, which contains the sperm* that might fertilise a women, stays inside the condom and cannot escape. So a condom prevents unwanted pregnancies.

The use of a condom at the same time protects both partners from contracting venereal diseases – STIs*, including HIV* – from each other, because all of these viruses and infections are transmitted through body fluids, such as semen and blood.

Why do some women insist that a condom be used during sex?

All women who wish to avoid pregnancy* or STIs should! Correctly used, a condom protects them from an unwanted pregnancy and against STIs, and especially prevents them contracting the HIV virus. For these reasons a woman may insist that her partner or husband uses a condom to protect herself. It is her right to do so.

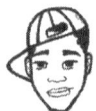

Are condoms really safe?

They are not always 100% safe, but condoms are much, much safer than having unprotected sex. The reason why no contraceptive is entirely safe is because they must be used correctly to be effective and people sometimes make mistakes. Condoms don't tear easily, so if there is a mishap it is almost always because the condom was not used properly.

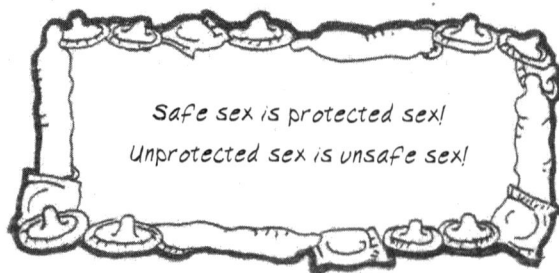

Safe sex is protected sex!
Unprotected sex is unsafe sex!

How does one use a condom correctly?

Always use a new and clean condom. The rolled-up sheath must be fitted over the head of the penis* and unrolled to cover it before sexual intercourse. Never use condoms with an oil-based lubricant (a gel or cream, e.g. Vaseline) because it will dissolve the condom and cause it to break. Water-based lubricants (such as KY gel) are safe. To be effective a condom must be fitted properly each time, and it must be used every single time you have sex. If you use a condom only four times out of five you still put yourself and your partner at risk.

Where does one find condoms?

Because of the danger of AIDS* one can find condoms all over the place today – in health clinics and hospitals, where they are usually handed out free, or you can buy them from chemists and pharmacies, supermarkets and even from street vendors and slot machines in pubs, hotels and restaurants. Some NGOs too distribute condoms free of charge. If you need one urgently, don't forget that your friends might have some in stock.

Can condoms damage my penis if I use them regularly?

No. Condoms do not cause any damage if worn properly, unless you have an allergic reaction to latex rubber. If this is the case you should look for a condom made from an alternate material, e.g. polyurethane.

Do all religions* approve of the use of condoms?

Some denominations, such as the Catholic Church, don't officially approve of the use of condoms, because they believe that sex should be practised only for procreation (the conceiving of children) and not for pleasure. People who are not married or do not want children, they say, should abstain from having sex.

Some people associate condoms with immoral behaviour, because they think that men who use condoms must be sleeping around with more than one partner. However, today the use of condoms is not a question of morality; it is a case of protecting your health and your life and that of your partner, and of preventing the making of unwanted babies.

Does using condoms lead to prostitution*?

No, most people who use condoms are not prostitutes and will never become sex workers*. There have always been sex workers – it is even said that prostitution is the oldest profession in the world. (By the way, remember that if men did not want to pay for sex there would be no prostitutes.) But today, more than ever before, sex workers and their clients need to be protected from STIs*, and condoms are the best way for them to protect themselves, their partners, as well as their partners' subsequent partners from the dangers of unprotected sex.

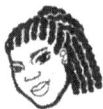

Why do some men refuse to use condoms?

Some men prefer to remain inside the woman's vagina* after ejaculation*, but because the semen might leak out of the condom, this shouldn't happen if you want to play it safe. Other men feel that condoms inhibit their sexual performance because they lose some of the sensation when they wear a condom during sex. Such men often say it is not manly to wear a condom or that 'it is like eating sweets with the wrapper on'. There are also men who associate condoms with infidelity (not being faithful*), and then there are some men who are simply too lazy or careless to bother about condoms and safe sex*. Most of these attitudes are strictly selfish, and give no thought to the other person, or for tomorrow.

If however a couple have a loving, faithful, monogamous relationship there is no reason for the man to wear a condom.

What are female condoms?

A female condom is like a male condom but larger. It is a loose polyurethane bag with an inner and an outer ring, worn by the woman inside her body. The bag is made of thinner material than a male condom and a man is less likely to object that he loses sensation during sex. But it takes some time to get used to a female condom, because it can be uncomfortable at first and it can also slip out of place. Health workers say that you should try them at least three times before you give up on them. In South Africa female condoms are available at pharmacies and some clinics, and in Zimbabwe through some NGOs, but they are expensive. They are generally not given out free.

Female condoms have the added advantage that they cover most of the woman's outer labia ('lips'), and so can protect her against STIs* and HIV* infection, even during foreplay* or heavy petting* when the penis* may come into contact with this sensitive area.

Contraception

Also see Family planning

Contraception is the general term used for the different methods and devices available to people who want to avoid pregnancies. The two main forms of contraception are total abstinence* and the use of some form of contraception. The most common methods of contraception are:

1. **Oral contraception**, commonly known as 'The Pill'. It is a tablet that a woman takes by mouth daily. The tablet stops the process of ovulation* (the monthly formation of ova• (eggs) in women's bodies, which, when fertilised by the man's sperm*, grow into babies). The advantage of this form of contraception is that it is almost 100% effective if used properly. One disadvantage is that the pills have to be taken daily to be effective, so a woman has to be responsible and disciplined to use 'The Pill' effectively. If tablets are forgotten or skipped, pregnancy* can occur. Another disadvantage is that contraceptive tablets change the hormones* in women's bodies, and this affects some women negatively: some put on weight, others become moody. However, the majority of women who use 'The Pill' remain healthy. 'The Pill' is the most common birth control* contraceptive used in southern Africa.

2. **Condoms*** (male). This is a rubber sheath that is placed over the penis* before having sexual intercourse*. The sheath prevents the man's semen from entering the woman's vagina* during sexual intercourse. In this way, pregnancy is avoided. The advantage of this form of contraceptive is that it is easily available and cheap, often free. A couple only needs to use it when taking part in sexual activity, so it does not affect or change the woman's body in any way. It also offers the added protection against HIV/AIDS* and other STIs*. A disadvantage is that the condom can tear. It also has to be fitted with proper care: the rolled-up sheath must be fitted over the head of the penis and rolled down to cover it before the beginning of sexual intercourse. Condoms must never be re-used.

3. **Intra-Uterine Device (IUD).** This device made of copper or synthetic fibre, also known as '**the coil**' or '**Copper T**', is placed inside the woman's womb (uterus)• by a doctor. It causes the uterus to expel anything that enters it. Therefore the egg is prevented from attaching itself in the uterus wall and developing into a foetus. In this way pregnancy• is avoided. The advantage of this form of contraceptive is that it is easy to manage, because once the IUD is fitted you can forget about it. Normally it is replaced every 3 or 4 years.

4. **Abstinence** (sexual)*. This method is used by some couples who do not altogether refrain from having sex at all times, but who only abstain from sex during the time of the month when the woman is most fertile (the time of ovulation) – 14 days after the start of a new menstrual cycle. By not having sexual intercourse during these days, the woman cannot fall pregnant. But be careful, because of individual variations in the likely days of ovulation this method is not always reliable.

5. **Injection** (birth control). This method of contraception is for women. There are two kinds of injection: Provera is injected every three months, and Nurestrate is given every two months. The injection is an effective contraceptive and is widely used and very popular. An advantage of this method is that women do not have to remember to take a pill daily, while a disadvantage is that the injection frequently disturbs menstruation* – but it usually returns to normal after a while. Fertility is not impaired permanently, but women should get advice at a clinic on the best type of injection to use, and they must receive the injection at the specified time.

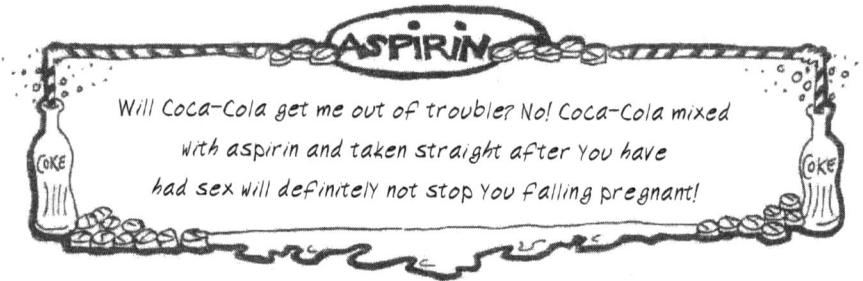

Will Coca-Cola get me out of trouble? No! Coca-Cola mixed with aspirin and taken straight after you have had sex will definitely not stop you falling pregnant!

How do I decide what form of contraception to use?
Each method of contraception has certain advantages and certain disadvantages. Choosing a contraceptive is a personal matter. Factors which may influence your decision are: your age, the state of your health, how active you are sexually, and whether you can take the risk of falling pregnant. The best is to visit a family planning clinic or a doctor, because they can advise you on the most suitable form of contraception for you.

Why are some religions* opposed to contraception?
Some churches, like the Catholics, are against all forms of contraception. Some priests think that it is it wrong for people to partake in sex for enjoyment, rather than for the procreation of children. However, the attitude of some priests in the Catholic church is more liberal in some places than others, usually because they recognise that the burden of poverty is increased with larger families, so some orthodox religious leaders are rethinking their position on the issue of contraception. They realise that if the use of contraceptives is not allowed, many unwanted children are born, often to poor parents* who cannot adequately provide for them; also the use of condoms* prevents the spread of the HIV* virus.

Do unmarried girls have access to contraceptives?
Yes, unmarried girls who are over the age of 18 years are legally entitled to access to all contraceptive methods. Girls under the age of 18 years

are required to have the consent of their parents*, however, although this age limit is not always enforced by family doctors.

Where can I go to obtain 'The Pill' or other contraceptives?
Contraceptives should be easily available at all local suburban and rural clinics, or through your family/local doctor. Condoms are often given free of charge but can also be purchased at any pharmacy.

How reliable is 'The Pill'?
You can rely on 'The Pill' to prevent pregnancy*, but for it be effective you have to take it daily and not skip some days. 'The Pill' is given on prescription, so before taking it you must consult a doctor or clinic sister.

Corporal punishment
Also see Child abuse

Corporal punishment is when a parent or teacher punishes a child by caning or hitting him or her. In South Africa corporal punishment is a criminal offence (punishable by law). In Zimbabwe a parent may legally discipline a child by hitting him or her, but if the child is injured, either physically or emotionally, it is also punishable by law. In both Zimbabwean and South African schools physical punishment (caning) is allowed only for boys, and must be done by the head of the school in the presence of another staff member, and any caning must be recorded.

Courtesy
Also see Manners

To be courteous is to be kind and polite in the way you act and to treat other people, young and old, with consideration.

Does courtesy have a place in today's society?
Certainly, even though courtesy or politeness is often considered an old-fashioned concept. Some people argue that everyone is equal, so why do we need to behave politely towards others? However, while some people think like this, being polite is simply thinking about the other person as well as oneself. A golden rule is: treat other people the way you would like them to treat you. Most people look favourably on a young person who stands up to offer a seat in the bus or train to an older or handicapped person,

or to a pregnant woman; or who acts politely in other ways, like helping someone with a heavy load or helping a stranger to push his or her car when the battery is flat.

Cross-dressing

Cross-dressing is when someone likes to dress in the clothes belonging to the opposite gender*. Cross-dressing does not mean you are homosexual* or want to change your sex. Many men get a thrill out of wearing women's clothes at home occasionally, but a true male cross-dresser wears women's clothes in public places and may pass himself off as a woman.

Aren't drag queens also men in women's clothes?

You have to distinguish between drag artists and drag queens. Drag artists are men in the entertainment world who wear women's clothes for public performances. One of the most famous drag artists comes from Australia: Dame Edna, who is a well-known comedienne known all over the English-speaking world. In South Africa, Pieter-Dirk Uys has created an equally famous female personality, Evita Bezuidenhout, who often makes her audiences laugh at local politicians and politics.

However, men in drag are not always involved in public entertainment. There are sometimes well-known, very vivacious, gay* men who wear women's clothes and make-up, often with great style, and are so well known within the gay community that they are called drag queens.

Are women who wear trousers* cross-dressers?

No, today many women throughout the world wear trousers as part of their everyday dress. In some communities, e.g. in Pakistan, loose trousers have always been worn by women. Some people still believe that it is inappropriate – but the role of women has changed over time and it has become practical and fashionable for women to wear slacks. And mostly the jeans and jackets that young people wear today – unisex dressing – is a statement about equality.

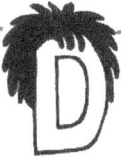

Dating

Also see **Faithfulness, Free love**

Dating – also sometimes called 'courting' or 'courtship' – is when two people who like and feel attracted to each other go out together and spend time together. There are two types of dating: casual dating, when you go out just as friends, and more serious dating, when you go out as girlfriend* and boyfriend* and where there is an understanding of commitment* between two people. A committed couple may be called 'an item' in some circles these days, while others call this kind of dating 'going steady'.

Two people can go on a date by themselves – to watch a movie or to go dancing – or they can go on a date in a group.

At what age should teenagers start dating?

There is no general rule in this regard. Usually a time arrives when girls and boys become aware of each other and like to spend time together. For some this happens in their early teens, for others much later. You need to ask yourself if you really want to go out with someone, or whether you feel you should simply because all your friends are dating. That is not a good enough reason! You should feel ready for dating, because with dating comes responsibilities. It is not always possible to know beforehand that your date will treat you the way you want to be treated, so you should feel sure of your principles and what you would allow and where you would draw the line.

It is always good to discuss your uncertainties with someone in your family, and to consider things such as: Is this guy a family friend? How long have I known him? What attracts me to him? It is a good sign if a first date is already based on trust, understanding and shared values.

How do I approach a girl for a date?

Asking a girl out on a date can be quite scary, especially if you are not sure what her response will be. Ask yourself why you want to date this particular girl. If you are not sure, wait until you know her a little better or until you feel that you have something to share with her. Remember that she is just as likely to be as nervous as you are, and that she might also feel more comfortable if you suggest something fairly low-key, such as going for a walk, studying together or going to a movie, which you can both enjoy without having to talk all the time. You can also do something together in a group, which will give you the opportunity to get to know each other a little better within a situation where you don't feel tense.

What does taking out a girl involve?

Taking a girl out on a first date can make one feel a bit tense and nervous, especially if you really like the person. So first wait for a good opportunity to ask her out and then do it in a way that would not put her off: not too serious but also not too casual, and suggest something specific, such as a film or a dance. If she has accepted, you need to plan: Where will you meet her? How are you getting wherever you're going – by taxi? Walking? By car? What can you afford? What will she enjoy? You might even ask her for ideas.

Before going to meet her for the date, make sure you have enough money on you. Then relax, be yourself and enjoy her company. Remember she would not have accepted your invitation if she didn't want to spend some time with you.

Who pays when two people go out on a date?

It is always good for the person who invited you on a first date to pay for the outing. Previously when a boy and a girl dated it was expected of him to carry on paying for everything. Times have changed, however, and once you begin to go out regularly it is natural to 'go Dutch'. This means that you each pay half, or that you take turns to pay.

Some dates can be quite expensive, for example eating out and watching a movie afterwards. In such a case it might be a good idea to pay for yourself. Unless he has lots of money don't take for granted that your partner will pay for you, and if you can afford it offer to help pay. Remember the way someone handles money – how generous, how careful or how fair they are – affects the way others regard that person.

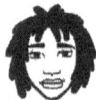

Who pays if the guy is very rich?

It is never a good idea for him to show off that he has a lot of money. It may work in the short term, but it won't in the long run. People will get irritated and fed-up with him.

A sugar-daddy is an older man who provides gifts and other luxuries to a much younger woman, usually as 'soft' payment for sexual favours. If an older man flatters you and offers you gifts, remember that there might be a very high price to pay.

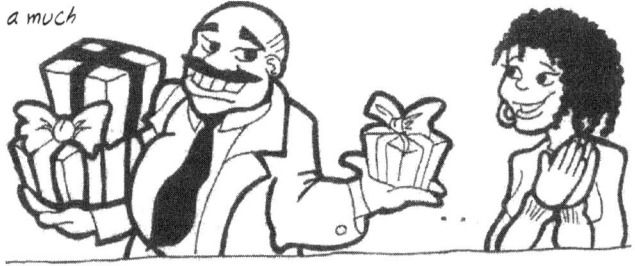

Should I go out with someone from a different culture to my own?

It is usually easier to get along with someone from your own background, but it is not impossible to get on equally well with someone from a completely different culture. Most societies share certain important basic principles, for example telling the truth, not stealing, caring for children and the elderly, and treating strangers with respect*. It is usually their religious beliefs that differ and their concept of God. This would influence the traditions and rituals around the key moments in a person's life: birth, coming of age, marriage* and death. But it might also influence attitudes to women, people of a different faith, nature and animals.

So, as long as you feel you can respect the other person's culture and beliefs and he respects yours, there is no reason why you should not go out with him. Learning about a different culture and sharing ideas about your own is usually exciting, but also challenging. It requires give and take. Don't expect to have everything your own way. Don't assume your culture is superior. Show respect for the other culture, but also demand respect for your own.

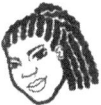

What should I do when I don't want to go on a date?

When you are invited out and you don't want to go, say no in a polite, honest manner. Try not to hurt the other person's feelings. And remember, saying no does not give you the right to gossip about it with your friends or to mock the person who has asked you out. If you do this you will get a reputation for being nasty and cruel. Try to imagine how you would feel if you were in the other person's position.

It is possible that you might like a person as a friend, but don't want to date him. Try to explain this to him, because it would be a pity to lose the friendship*. Honesty is very important. Don't mislead someone into believing that you will go out with him later if this is not true.

43

Why are girls attracted to older guys?

Girls tend to grow up faster than boys, so they sometimes find boys of their own age silly and childish and prefer older boys who are more adult. Often older boys or men are kinder, more mature, wiser and gentler. This makes them less demanding and selfish. On the other hand, some girls are attracted to older boys or grown-up men because they can offer them material things: expensive gifts, cash, cars and cell phones.

Why are some older men attracted to young girls?

Some older men with lots of money 'buy' young girls' attention because it makes them feel powerful and young themselves. They may have a wife of their own age in whom they now have little sexual interest. Girls should be careful of such men: some like the idea of having sex with a virgin. It makes them feel special, but some also believe that it is safer to have sex with a girl who has never slept with a man before, and some even believe that this can cure them of AIDS*. Men like these do not care about the girl at all, only about their own selfish desires.

Can I date more than one girl at a time?

It is good to have fun and find out about other people when you are a teenager. So light-hearted but caring friendships that are open, warm and honest and which involve taking different girls out to parties, or to see a film or to a dance, are a good idea. But only as long as you are honest about your intentions and the girls understand the situation.

If you are regularly dating one girl and you still want to date other girls as well, it is important to talk to her about your feelings and needs. Remember you have to respect* her feelings and needs too. So you and she may perhaps decide together that it is fine for you both to date other people. If, however, you and your girlfriend* decided that you are only going to date each other, then you have made some form of commitment*. Most people say that it is difficult to be emotionally involved with more than one person at the same time. The key to your question is: how honest you are with your girlfriend and with yourself?

Remember if you are in a sexual relationship with the girl you are dating, it is important to practise safe sex*. And if you are dating and having sex with more than one partner you are putting yourself as well as all of them at risk of contracting STIs* or HIV*. You should be extra-responsible about the use of condoms*.

What about being alone with a guy in a secluded place?

Never be alone with someone you don't trust. The most important question to ask yourself is: Do I feel safe with this guy? When one first begins to date a guy you may not know him well enough to want to be alone with him. If you feel like this, but you still want to get to know him better, rather suggest that you do something social together and make sure you go somewhere where you know other people.

Some parents* don't find it acceptable for a girl and a boy to be alone together. It is never a good idea to do something behind your parents' back, but if you know this is going to happen and you don't want to tell them it would be sensible for you to tell a trusted friend or another adult where you will be. This is for your own safety, in case something goes wrong. Then someone will know where and with whom you are.

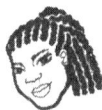

When should I break off a relationship?

There is no easy answer – some relationships last long, others not. But considering the following questions might lead you to an answer: Do I feel happy and secure in this relationship? Is it possible to discuss something that bothers me about our relationship with my partner? Is he interested in solving the problem and improving the situation? If all the answers are 'no', you should seriously reconsider the relationship. What is the point of going out with someone if it doesn't make you feel happy and safe? Who you can't talk to? Can't share your worries with? Can't have fun with?

If a relationship has become abusive* in any way, whether physically, sexually, emotionally, or verbally, you need to stand back and ask yourself whether it is healthy or safe to continue with it.

Is it acceptable for a girl to say 'I love you' first?

A girl's confidence to say 'I love you' first may be influenced by her cultural or religious background. However, owing to the spread of democracy and the influence of the women's liberation movement – which has fought hard for women's voices to be heard – ideas about the equality of the genders are now widely accepted, and a woman should feel confident to say what she thinks and know that her ideas are as important as anyone else's.

If you feel you want to say 'I love you' first, why not say it? To be told that you are loved is a wonderful thing. For men too! The only problem is if you are unsure how the boy will respond to this declaration you may risk rejection or ridicule. Sometimes it is better to fall back on the old rule: WHEN IN DOUBT, DON'T.

A person with 'agency' is someone who is confident about what they are doing and pro-active in their approach. These days we would say they are 'empowered' when it comes to sex.

How do I decide whether or not to have sex with my boyfriend*?

This is a complicated matter. Since contraception* has become freely available and the idea of sex before marriage – 'free love'* – widely accepted, great emphasis has been put on the sexual aspect of a relationship. This has resulted in peer pressure* being put on young people to be sexually active. Often girls in particular are told: 'If you love me you will have sex with me. If you refuse it shows you don't love me.' This is intimidation, because you may fear that if you say 'no' your boyfriend will break off the relationship. You may also fear that your peers will make fun of you and call you 'old-fashioned' or 'prudish' because you have said no.

If your boyfriend would like you two to have a sexual relationship and you do not feel ready for it you should discuss your feelings with him, and if he really cares for you he will respect your decision. If there is open communication and mutual respect* in a relationship it is possible to survive without sex.

How should one dress for a date?

How one dresses is a personal choice: it will depend on the occasion, the level of formality and what you have in your wardrobe. If you are invited somewhere that you have not been before, find out beforehand what kind of place it is. You won't want to be wearing high heels on a picnic!

What you wear and how you wear your clothes will reflect your taste and say something about the type of person you are. If, for example, you wear very skimpy clothes a guy may assume you are sexually confident, and this is how he will treat you.

Generally speaking, women dress up more than men do, because they are more into clothing than men. However, if you like dressing smartly and the guy could not care less what he looks like you should ask yourself if you should dress more informally, or suggest that he dresses better. But remember what you wear is usually a reflection of your values and if you disagree profoundly with a guy over clothes you need to consider how much you really have in common.

Should one forget about a girl who is already dating someone else?

Everyone should be allowed to express how they feel about someone else, but to break up someone else's relationship is generally wrong. However, quietly telling the girl that you care for her and respect her decision to be with the other guy is acceptable. Joking with the man and telling him what a lucky fellow he is is another way of communicating your feelings.

Don't become obsessed about a girl who is committed* to someone else. It often happens that one person loves another with whom he or she can never have a relationship. It is sad and frustrating, but do not dream about what is impossible. You are likely to find another person to love and admire.

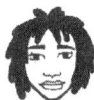

Will having lots of money make me attractive to girls?

Unfortunately the media – advertising, television, radio, magazines, movies – often create the impression that money makes you successful and that if a man is rich he will be popular and attractive to women. This is not always true in real life. People may use material wealth as symbols of status and power, but their money will not ensure that they are loved, liked or respected. If a girl is attracted to someone only because he has money, she loves his money and not him and she is only interested in what he can buy her. On the other hand, if you are fun to be with, caring and easy to talk to, you will find that people, girls too, are attracted to you whether you have lots of money or not.

Depression

Depression is an intense sense of sadness or loss. Depressed people often feel lonely, and they lose their enthusiasm for life and for relationships with other people. The feeling of depression can be described as a cold feeling of dread, sometimes accompanied by bad dreams, or the tendency to snap. Depressed people often feel overwhelmed by small problems, or issues that appear to be much bigger than they really are. Sometimes there are real reasons why someone feels miserable, for example, grief* about a loved one who has died, or about a meaningful relationship that has come to an end. Someone can also feel miserable and sad about failing an exam or not having a job. However, if the sense of sadness becomes so overwhelming that it affects how you experience other aspects of life it has become depression. A depressed person often feels like a failure, and his or her whole identity becomes threatened. Seriously depressed people stand a better chance of recovery if they receive counselling. In some people depression stems from a chemical imbalance which can be corrected by medication.

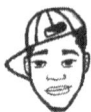

My girlfriend* seems to be crying constantly for no reason. Is she depressed?

Depression is often accompanied by a sudden inexplicable desire to cry. Try to talk about it to her and find out what makes her feel so unhappy. If she can't tell you and you remain worried about her state of mind, encourage her to see a counsellor or to speak to a doctor or someone at her church that she trusts.

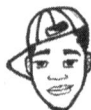

What can I do to overcome depression?

Firstly, try to identify the source of the feeling. What is causing this sadness? What are the reasons behind it? Discuss your misery or anxieties with a close friend. With discussion you will often find that you understand your own feelings better. If possible try to see a counsellor, someone who has been professionally trained to help one work out ways to overcome depression.

I often think I am worthless. Does that mean I suffer from depression?

Try to work out why you feel this way. The best thing you can do is to talk to someone close to you and try to analyse your feelings and your experiences. Putting things into words could give you a new perspective and help you to see things differently. Can you truly say about yourself that you have no value as a human being? You could be experiencing these feelings because you're comparing yourself to other people, wanting or trying to be someone you're not. Learning to understand yourself means recognising your strengths and limits and accepting them.

What is the difference between anxiety and depression?

Anxiety and depression are two different states of mind, but there is a definite link between the two. We can feel anxious about many things, e.g. family problems, being bullied or teased by someone who seems sharper or more intelligent than we are, failing an exam. Feeling a little anxious or nervous is natural, it happens to everyone. But if your anxieties persist, and if they start affecting your sleep and appetite for food, you are probably depressed. This type of anxiety is often caused by setting unattainable standards or goals for yourself. It may also have to do with what you think someone expects of you, or how you think society will judge you.

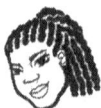

What can I do to overcome anxiety?

Firstly ask yourself: Are these fears real, or are they imagined? Counselling or at least discussing these feelings with a friend will help you to work through this question.

Is it true that teenagers become more easily depressed than adults?
When you are an adolescent your body undergoes a lot of change. These hormonal* changes can contribute to mood swings: one moment you might feel great, and then suddenly miserable. As a teenager you are constantly discovering things about yourself and this can cause feelings of isolation and insecurity. This does not necessarily mean you are depressed. However, if these feelings start to overwhelm you and it feels as if your whole life is out of control, try to get professional help.

Don't trap yourself into believing:

> I don't feel good, therefore I am bad. Therefore no one loves me

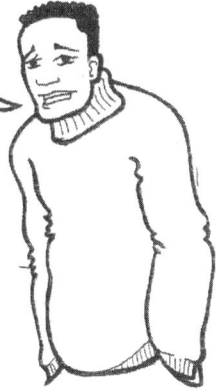

My cousin committed suicide*. Was he depressed?
Probably. People who commit suicide have given up on life, often because of a deep sense of despair, failure, hopelessness or loss of control. All these are characteristics of a depressed state of mind. So if ever someone you know seems to be experiencing these feelings, she or he might feel suicidal – give them as much love* as you can, but also try to persuade them to see a counsellor. Sometimes they may need extra guidance and support to help them get through a particularly difficult situation, and this can best be given by professionals. Samaritans in Zimbabwe and Life Line in South Africa are organisations which can be phoned at any time of the day or night and are there to help people who are feeling depressed.

Diet

The term 'diet' means the combination of foods that one eats to produce a specific result, e.g. to stay healthy, or to lose weight, or to get rid of an allergy, or to control diabetes. Many people, however, use the word as a verb – to diet – and then it is limited to meaning 'to eat in such a way as to lose weight'.

What is a healthy, balanced diet?
A general guideline is that your daily diet should consist of
    50% carbohydrates (starch),
    30% fruit and vegetables and
    20% protein.

Men normally need to eat more than women; people who do physical work need more food than people doing an office job, and growing children need more food than grown-ups, so depending on these factors, your daily intake should be

between 6 and 11 servings of carbohydrates
>   One serving = 1 slice of bread, or
>   2 to 3 tablespoons of rice or samp, or sadza, or
>   1 medium-size potato or sweet potato
+ *5 servings of fruit and vegetables,* especially green and orange and red ones
>   One serving = 1 fruit or a medium cup of vegetables
+ *1 to 2 servings of protein* – fish, meat, soya beans, or an egg
>   One serving = 200 to 250 g.

Is it true that some cooking methods are healthier than others?

Yes. Raw food (except meat, of course) is healthier than cooked food, because heat destroys many of the vitamins and minerals found in fresh food.

But if you don't want to eat raw vegetables, steam them rather than boil them in lots of water for a long time, because the nutrients (vitamins and minerals) that aren't destroyed by the heat will end up in the water.

When it comes to meat it is better to grill or braai (barbecue) it than to fry it in oil or fat, because fat is very unhealthy.

Are some types of food unhealthy to eat?

Most certainly! Sugary foods such as biscuits, cakes, sweets, chocolates, fizzy drinks, lots of sugar in tea or coffee, etc., are bad for you. Too much sugar in your diet causes tooth cavities and also obesity[*] because too much sugar intake produces more energy than your body can burn up.

Fatty foods such as fast foods (hamburgers, fish and chips) and food fried in oil or covered with rich sauces also cause obesity, because fat gets absorbed by the body very easily.

Other foods that you should try to cut out of your diet as far as possible are: refined foods (e.g. white bread and white sugar) and processed foods (canned foods, processed cheeses and meats, such as polony). The more refined and processed food is, the more chemicals are needed to preserve them, and chemicals are not good for the body. For this reason it is advisable to: EAT AS MUCH FRESH AND UNREFINED FOODS AS POSSIBLE.

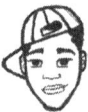

Are some meals more important than others?

Yes, breakfast is by far the most important meal of the day, because it regulates your metabolism (all the processes that occur in your body, resulting in growth, the production of energy and getting rid of waste material) for the rest of the day. Also, five smaller meals are better than two or three large ones, because the regular intake of food keeps your body functioning at a regular pace: breakfast between 7 and 8 in the morning, a mid-morning snack between 10 and 11 a.m., lunch between 12 and 1 p.m., an afternoon snack around 3 or 4 p.m., and the evening meal at 6 or 7 p.m. It is not good to eat of lot of food just before you go to bed.

It is also bad to eat just before you do heavy exercise, because blood is needed by both your digestive system and your muscles!

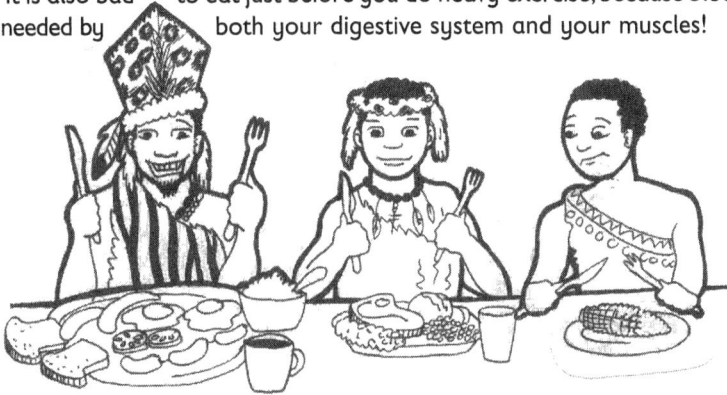

Breakfast like a king   lunch like a prince   dine like a pauper

Divorce

A couple who divorce have their marriage* legally dissolved.

Why do some parents* get divorced?
There isn't a single reason for this sad decision. Some couples get married when they are young and before they really know themselves or each other. Only later they discover that they have misjudged the other person, that they actually do not love their partner and don't want to be with him or her for the rest of their lives. Some couples have children before they are ready for the responsibility and feel that children tie them down and do not allow them to do the things they wanted to do. Often one parent blames the other for his or her unhappiness because they did not discuss beforehand whether they wanted children, and how children would affect their lives. When a married couple start having children too soon it often increases the tension between them and leads to a divorce.

A 'forced' marriage because of an unplanned pregnancy* can be another reason for parents getting divorced. Sometimes such a marriage is the result of just one sexual experience without contraception*. If the couple hardly knew each other when this happened, you can imagine that it is unlikely that they will be suited as marriage partners.

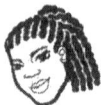

Why do people who are unhappily married decide to have a baby?
Some couples do this because they hope that children will hold their marriage together. They hope that a baby that they both care for will make them grow closer and love each other again. However, if their relationship has already begun to go wrong this seldom works.

How does one cope with divorced parents*?
The best thing to do if you are in this unhappy situation is to try to make friends of your own outside the family circle that can provide you with extra support and affection. Also try to develop relationships with other adults whom you trust and can talk to. Try not to take sides and to understand what went wrong between your parents, so you can learn from their mistakes and not repeat them. Remember you and your siblings, if you have any, are not responsible for the break-up so you need not feel guilty about it.

Why do divorced parents often neglect their children?
A divorce is usually an extremely difficult time for the entire family and everyone must adjust to many drastic changes. Sometimes the children get caught in the middle, with each parent feeling that the main responsibility for childcare lies with the other.

Both parents may be angry, sad, bitter and worried. They are experiencing the destruction of a dream, and the failed relationship often makes them feel guilty and inadequate. All these emotions are difficult to deal with, even for an adult. Sometimes one parent might have fallen in love with someone else. This might cause him or her emotional distress and feelings of guilt which could take the parent's attention away from the children. The father or mother might be so in love that the new relationship gets all the attention that used to be given to their offspring.

What can one do if you feel that your divorced parent is neglecting you?
The best thing to do is to talk to a sympathetic adult whom you trust. Try to explain to him or her how you feel. Talking things over always makes one feel better because it helps you sort out your thoughts and feelings, and get the anxieties off your chest. Once the situation has calmed down, and your parents are feeling less upset themselves, you may be able to talk to each of them yourself and explain how hard it has been for you. Most parents care very deeply for their children and would appreciate the opportunity to have a heart to heart talk about the thing that has disrupted all of your lives. Like you, parents are human and have shortcomings, and dur-

ing a divorce they can get so caught up in their emotions that it might look as if they have forgotten or no longer love their children. It is seldom the case.

Why would a couple who do not have children get divorced?

In some traditional societies children are a sign of status and prosperity, so people who do not have children are often looked down on. In some families it is particularly important for a man to produce an heir, someone who can inherit the family wealth and carry on the family name. If it turns out that the wife of such a man will never be able to produce a baby because of infertility*, he may feel he should divorce her and take another wife who can give him children. People often assume that the wife must be the infertile member of the couple, but the husband may, of course, be the infertile one ... A couple can have tests to see which is infertile, and whether anything can be done about it.

However, this question assumes that the only reason for a couple to marry is to have children. Many couples these days decide that they do not want children. They are together because they love each other, enjoy each other's company, respect each other's values and are in some ways each other's best friend.

Domestic violence see Abuse

Drugs

Drugs is a general term used for chemical or herbal substances which when used by people alter the state of mind and bodily sensations of the user. Some drugs (often called 'recreational drugs' because they are not used medicinally) are stimulants that excite and increase feelings and sensations, such as LSD and ecstasy. Other drugs are relaxants that make people sleepy and lazy, such as dagga – mbanje.

Many people think drugs are harmless and only give you pleasure, but all too often drugs cause enormous misery. The effect of drugs varies from person to person, but in the end drug use invariably leads to problems. Most drugs are habit-forming, so people become psychologically or physically addicted to them, and if they can't find or afford to buy the drug will do anything in order to find it to get the 'kick' they've become used to, or the 'fix' that their bodies desperately need. Selling and buying drugs are illegal in all the countries in southern Africa, as is the possession of drugs, and offenders are punishable by law.

Remember that drugs that have to be injected, such as heroin and morphine, cause a further risk because if a new needle is not used there is a danger of being infected with the HIV* virus.

Coffee is addictive too. Can you call it a drug as well?

Yes, strictly speaking coffee is a drug because it contains a chemical called caffeine, which is a stimulant. But generally the term 'drugs' refers to narcotic drugs – drugs that alter your mental and psychological state, change your behaviour and can cause serious bodily harm, and even kill you if an overdose is taken. Even excessive amounts of caffeine – too many strong coffees – can have unpleasant effects.

What is meant by 'soft drugs'?

Soft drugs are drugs such as *mbanje* or *dagga* (also known as marijuana and ganja, amongst others) and recreational drugs such as poppers, used to alter your mood and put you in a 'party mood'. Unlike 'hard drugs' (cocaine, heroin, mandrax, crack), the use of soft drugs on their own does not lead to the physical addiction* which causes serious withdrawal symptoms if you stop taking them. Soft drugs can lead to a mental or psychological dependency.

Soft drugs also do not have such a dramatic effect as hard drugs. But the use of soft drugs is dangerous in that it often leads to the use of hard drugs, because once you are involved with drugs, and with the people who use them, you easily move from one drug to another in search of new sensations. So, better avoid all drugs – soft or hard!

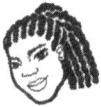

Many of my friends say drugs are cool and that I should try them just once.

Don't. Drugs are expensive, illegal, dangerous, addictive, and in some cases cause anti-social behaviour. Once you have started using drugs and are mixed up with people who take them regularly it is difficult to break away again. Teenagers are often under pressure to experiment, whether it is with alcohol* or cigarettes* or with a drug, because they are told it is a 'cool' and 'mind-expanding' experience. Don't be tempted. Most young people end up feeling rotten after taking drugs, and if it becomes a habit they start behaving badly, spend lots of money, lose their friends who do not take drugs and their performance at school and on the sportsfield suffers.

Moreover, if you become an addict, i.e. dependent on a drug which costs a great deal of money (recreational drugs are not cheap), then this can lead to crime.

How can I help my boyfriend* to stop taking drugs?

The first step is to get your boyfriend to admit that he has a drug problem and that he needs help in order to stop. There are a number of organisations that specifically help people with drug problems. Identify one near to you and encourage your boyfriend to go there for help. Or speak to an adult you trust.

How can you tell if someone is taking drugs?

If he or she is smoking dagga, their eyes may appear red or dazed. People who use other drugs may experience mood swings and they may also be withdrawn and quiet, and find it difficult to concentrate for long. But a surer indication is if someone hangs around with a group of people who you know take drugs and know where to buy them.

Tackling the issue of drug use in your circle of friends is tricky and difficult, and can even be dangerous. It will be better to get help from a responsible adult like a school counsellor or a sympathetic teacher.

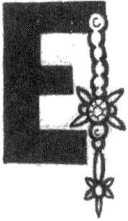

Education

The demands on society and on individual people have completely changed from the time when mankind lived in harmony with nature and survived as hunters and gatherers who needed no formal education. Today education opens up more opportunities to young people, makes them better informed, presents them with more choices and gives them more control over their lives. Someone who has not finished at least high school unfortunately has very limited chances of finding a good and well-paid job.

I keep thinking of my girlfriend* and can't concentrate on my studies!

Remind yourself that you don't have to do everything at once. Some of the best things in life are worth waiting for. Everyone needs to learn discipline. There are many distractions at school and at home. The best way to cope with this is to set aside a specific time for work and a specific time for pleasurable activities, and to stick to this routine. Regard your time for pleasure as a reward for having done your schoolwork.

It is a good sign that you are worried about your studies! If you are serious about being successful you will in any case not really enjoy yourself if you know your homework is not finished. Remember that you are preparing yourself for a good life: if you fail your exams now you might not be able to have the kind of job later that would make it possible for you to have the fun you dream about now.

Ejaculation

Ejaculation is what happens at the moment of orgasm* when a man has a sexual climax. At that moment semen is discharged from his erect penis*. When people talk informally they call this 'coming'.

Emotional abuse see Abuse

Escort

In terms of the law, an escort is someone who is hired to go to a party or provide company to a lonely person, usually in the evening. The escort is paid for her or his services. In reality the expectation is that an escort will have sex with the client and this is what is being paid for. In many countries, like the countries in southern Africa where prostitution* is illegal, so-called escort agencies get around the problem by offering escorts to their customers. An escort is therefore often a sex worker.*

My cousin says he wants to escort me when I go out. What does he mean?
Your cousin is offering you his protection, like a bodyguard. He wants to protect you from men who might make a nuisance of themselves. That could be very useful in certain social circumstances, such as at a club or a bar full of strangers! He clearly does not have the other kind of escorting in mind.

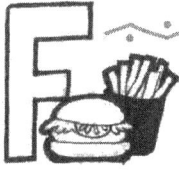

Faithfulness

Faithfulness – being faithful – in a relationship means that you are committed* to one person, or if you are a polygamist being faithful to your wives. It means you have chosen to date only your partner and not anyone else. Being faithful implies that you will have only one sexual partner at a time.

How can I get my girlfriend* to trust me and believe that I'm faithful?
If she doesn't trust you try to put yourself in her shoes and ask yourself why. Can you honestly say that she has no reason to doubt your honesty?

If you are honest about your own feelings and if you are respectful of your girlfriend's feelings and respond to her needs, she will learn to trust you. If you have made a mistake by neglecting her or spending too much time with another woman, accept some responsibility for what has happened. Never be afraid to say you are sorry, but never try to make excuses. Don't be dishonest.

If your girlfriend still doesn't trust you, she might have had some very bad past experiences and you will have to be very patient and understanding. If that doesn't work either, you might have to accept that things are never going to work out between you two and suggest that you break up.

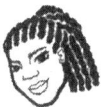

How do I know whether my boyfriend* is being unfaithful to me or not?
If he is constantly late for appointments or if he is vague about his movements the chances are that he is not being faithful. Try to ask him directly or to find out in some other way whether he is lying to you. If he is being unfaithful you need to make up your mind whether you want to stay with him, especially considering the dangers of HIV/AIDS*. However, remember that nagging, suspicion, constant questioning or accusations, not believing what he tells you and a lack of trust and understanding can ruin a relationship and drive someone away.

Why are some men such compulsive womanisers?
Usually such a man is afraid of accepting responsibility for himself and for others. He therefore chooses not to commit to any one person perma-

nently and rather to go out with a number of women so no one can lay claims to him. Many womanisers are men who are trying to prove their masculinity to themselves and to others.

What makes lovers unfaithful?
Lovers sometimes become unfaithful if they feel neglected, bored or ignored, or if they are not satisfied sexually. So they look out for other partners to satisfy these needs in their lives. If there is a problem or misunderstanding in a relationship and one of the partners refuses to talk about it the other one might look for comfort somewhere else. In some cases the man just wants to have many women in line because he finds it exciting to cheat on his partner, or because he wants to show off to impress friends with his 'power' over women. Quite often you hear men say that sex is a biological need and that once aroused, like hunger, it must be satisfied. They say that they need variety or that their wives don't give them enough sex. That is of course their excuse for being unfaithful.

Family planning

Also see **Birth control, Contraception**

In practical terms this means taking a decision about how many children you want and how many years you would like between each child. Effective family planning makes use of contraception*. Most towns and cities provide family-planning centres where couples can register and get advice on the most suitable method of contraception. There may be a small fee to pay, but usually the advice and the contraceptives are given free of charge. Medical doctors and health clinics provide the same service.

What is the point of family planning?
Successful family life is based on good planning. This means asking questions such as: How many children will we be able to provide for? What sort of education* should they get? How can we make sure that they get the best opportunities?

Thinking carefully about how many children you want, and planning for them, helps to ensure that you will be able to give them love*, attention, education and provide for their material needs.

Also, family planning makes it possible for a woman to decide if and when she will have children, and how many. In addition, it safeguards the long-term health of the woman because she does not have to strain her body by having too many children in quick succession.

Do women need to choose between children and work?

Not really. Many women who have jobs cannot care for their children full-time and employ a day-mother or leave their toddlers in the care of a crèche. If a woman can't afford this extra help it often means that she is overburdened by raising children and having to work at the same time. This is all the more reason for couples to plan carefully when to have a baby, so that it happens when the mother can cope with the dual responsibilities or afford help.

Single mothers* have an even greater problem. They have no partner with whom they can share the financial and emotional and childcare responsibilities – and the joys – of parenthood.

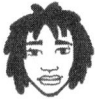

Are all employers willing to appoint young mothers?

Some employers are sympathetic towards women with small children. Besides not minding a woman taking the compulsory maternity leave when her baby is born, some employers even provide a crèche on their premises. However, other employers are hesitant to appoint young married women for fear that they might have a baby, which will interrupt their work. They also consider the care of a small child as the mother's own personal problem.

What is maternity leave?

It is the period of time to which a pregnant working woman is entitled by law to be away from work to give birth to a baby. South African labour law determines that no employer can fire a woman because she falls pregnant, and that on an average she should receive at least four months' maternity leave with full payment of her salary. In Zimbabwe a woman receives three months' leave on full pay. She may decide when she takes it. And there is now redress against employers who dismiss women when they become pregnant.

In some countries in Europe men share the responsibility for child care and are given paternity* leave. Some South African companies also allow their employees paternity leave.

Why was family planning less important in traditional societies?

In the olden days, before the industrial revolution, societies functioned with fewer pressures. The cost of having children and looking after them was not as high as today. In fact it was essential to have large families, because children provided the workforce and assurance that their parents would be cared for when they became old and helpless. At that time people did not have access to contraception*, but it was not so necessary, because many children died from disease, people did not grow very old, and women in particular died at a much younger age, worn out by childbirth* and family cares.

Today the world is faced with overpopulation and poverty, so it is very important not to have more children than you want and are able to care for properly. Unlike in olden times it is necessary to plan your family so that you do not put yourself under undue financial or emotional pressure.

Fatherhood

Another word for 'fatherhood' is 'paternity'. In the same way 'motherhood' is also known as 'maternity'.

What happens if you father a child while you're still at school?
If you become a father while you are in high school, you'll find yourself with many more responsibilities than other students of your age. In order to cope, you'll have to be very mature and responsible. Because it is important to finish your schooling and get a good education*, you shouldn't consider giving up your studies. On the other hand, as father you'll need to help support your baby's mother – either financially or by helping to care for the baby – even if you are no longer in a relationship with her.

How can you help the mother of your baby if you're studying?
You can assist her by offering to look after the baby after school. You can also contribute food, baby clothes and toys, and it is very important to take an active interest in the baby's health and development. If you are not able to do any of these things you could ask your mother or an older relative or family friend for help. It shows strength of character to take on the responsibilities of being a father, even if you have become a parent at a much younger age than you were planning to do.

What are the responsibilities of an unmarried father?
Legally, the father of a child has a duty to contribute to the maintenance of the child, even if he is not married to the mother. If he refuses, the child's mother can get a court order that forces him to pay. If he is working, the court order can stipulate that the money be deducted from his salary. However, the father has no automatic right to visit the child. If the mother refuses to let him see the child he may make an application in court, but the court will only allow this if they think it will be good for the child.

If possible, the father should build a relationship with his child by doing things together with him or her. Whether or not the father is still seeing the mother, he should try to come to an agreement with her about how he would like the child to be brought up. An unmarried father should never make it harder for the mother to raise the baby – especially in the beginning when she will be struggling on her own to cope with interrupted sleep, dirty nappies and visits to the clinic. He should rather, in whatever way possible, support the mother. It is in the interests of the child.

What are the legal consequences of a man fathering a child?

Whether or not the father of a child is married to its mother, there is a legal obligation on him to assist the mother with financial support. A court decides on the sum of money and how regularly it must be paid. A father who does not pay maintenance can be charged in a court of law.

What can a woman do if a man refuses to admit that he is the father of her child?

She can take the matter to court. The magistrate will probably order that a paternity* test (usually a blood test) be done that will prove whether or not the man is the child's father.

Feminism

Feminism advocates that women should enjoy the same social, political and economic rights as men and that women and men should be equal before the law. The feminist movement was very important in making women aware of inequalities on grounds of gender* and empowering women to develop their strengths.

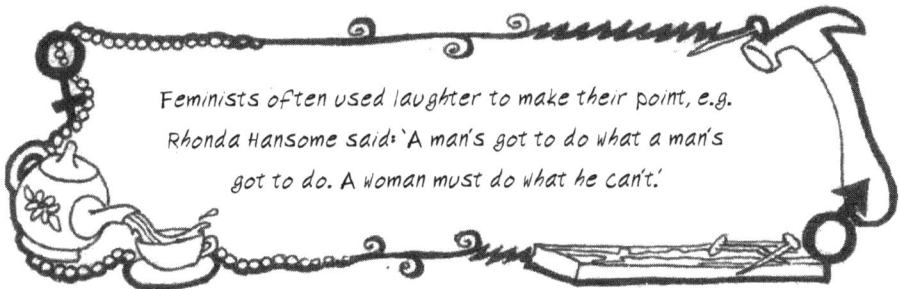

> Feminists often used laughter to make their point, e.g.
> Rhonda Hansome said: 'A man's got to do what a man's got to do. A woman must do what he can't.'

Flirting

Flirting is light-hearted behaviour intended to attract the attention of a member of the opposite sex, or in the case of gay* men and women, people of the same sex.

Is it wrong to flirt?
If both parties are flirting and you know it is just fun, it is harmless. It is a natural part of showing someone that you are attracted to them. However, if someone is deliberately flirting with someone much younger or more vulnerable without any intention of taking the relationship further in any way, flirting can send out the wrong messages and be confusing. Women who flirt with men in order to get them to buy them drinks or something else risk being called 'a tease', and some men might turn aggressive if they feel they have been given false promises by the woman.

Foreplay

Foreplay is what normally happens before two people engage in actual sexual intercourse*. Foreplay ranges from intense kissing* to mutual stroking and fondling of private parts (genitals). It is an important part of sexual interaction between people. It reinforces feelings of warmth and intimacy between couples, as opposed to just rushing to complete the sexual act. Women generally need more foreplay than men do to prepare them for sexual intercourse. A caring partner takes time to find out what feels good for his or her partner.

Free love

The idea of 'free love' was originally advocated in the hippie era of the Sixties, but it has influenced the current attitude that one can love freely without having to make a commitment* for life. People who believe in free love argue that sex is a natural, enjoyable part of life and that one doesn't have to stick to one sexual partner. They also say that people who have practised free love and have had several sexual partners are more mature when they eventually decide to commit themselves to one partner. Another argument for having more sexual experience is that it helps one make a better-informed decision about a life partner. In one sense free love is the same as 'pre-marital sex'.

However, relationships based on free love need discussion and agreement about the limits. On the positive side they can work in that affairs with other partners are not seen as a threat and a primary relationship can survive. But one partner may have more affairs than the other, which may lead to jealousy*, or what is seen as a 'one-night stand* may turn into something more serious, and undermine the primary relationship. The important thing to remember about free love is that it is supposed to be an arrangement based on mutual agreement and not on deception.

What are the pros and cons of sex before marriage?

Pre-marital sex gives a couple the opportunity to find out whether they are sexually compatible or not, in other words whether they can be happy with each other sexually and can fulfil each other's sexual needs. If two people discover only after their wedding* that that they are not sexually compatible it normally puts a strain on their marriage*. In this respect pre-marital sex seems sensible, providing that the two people love* and respect* each other.

However, most religions* do not approve of pre-marital sex, and if it is against someone's religious principles he or she should abstain* from sex and not feel pressured to be swayed by this argument.

Finally, pre-marital sex should only happen between two consenting adults who have taken precautions against having an unwanted child and the danger of HIV/AIDS*.

Does free love work for people?

Most people realise that any kind of 'love' involves two people and that having sex is an intimate relationship that cannot be treated lightly or irresponsibly. Therefore free love cannot fulfil people's real needs. Also, because of the spread of the HIV virus and other sexually transmitted diseases, people realise that it is much safer to have only one sexual partner and to practise safe sex*.

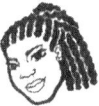

My sister's boyfriend* says he needs sex. Can this be true?

It is a common myth that guys 'need' to have sex. Sometimes guys use this myth to get sex. Guys do have higher testosterone* levels, which increases their sexual drive, but that isn't to say that they need to have sex. Women too have sexual desires. What we do with these drives is very important. If a guy does have a big sexual appetite he needs to find a safe way to feed that appetite, e.g. forming a trusting sexual relationship with a partner and engaging in safe sex, but that partner should consent. No one has the right to *demand* sex from someone else.

People can also release their sexual energy through masturbation*.

French kissing

French kissing is a sensual and intimate form of kissing where you put your tongue inside someone else's mouth and he or she puts his or her tongue in yours.

Can HIV* be spread through French kissing?
Normally the HIV virus cannot be transmitted through saliva – spit. If someone has a mouth or gum disease which causes a wound or bleeding, this can however present an exit or entry point for the virus. The tissue on the inside of the cheek, even of a healthy person, is particularly sensitive and can at times present an exit or entry point for the virus. French kissing should therefore be practised with caution.

Friendship

Friendship between two people is based on a genuine liking and not on mutual sexual attraction*.

How do I know who are my true friends?
A true friend is someone who you feel safe and comfortable with, someone you can trust For example, if you share your feelings and thoughts with a true friend he or she will listen and understand and respect* what you have to say, whereas someone who is not a true friend may make fun of you, and tell others what you told him or her in confidence. A true friend is someone who accepts you the way you are without trying to change you, and who will be supportive and helpful when you need support or help.

Should I tell a good friend that I love her?
You need to think carefully about whether it is wise to tell your friend that you love her. Being honest about your feelings is never wrong, but in this situation you may risk being hurt or rejected unless you suspect that she likes you in a special way too. If you have a very good friendship you may want to keep it that way and not make your friend feel uncomfortable by telling her about your loving feelings for her. On the other hand, it is very likely that a relationship that develops from a friendship will succeed, because the two people already know and trust one another. It is of course possible to feel love – great fondness – for a friend of either sex, without having a sexual interest in that friend.

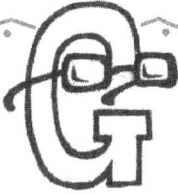

Gay

Also see **Homosexuality**

'Gay' is probably the term most frequently used today to refer to a homosexual person – in other words a person who prefers to have an intimate relationship with someone of his or her own sex instead of with someone of the opposite sex. Gay can refer to both men and women, but it usually refers to men while the word 'lesbian' is used to refer to women.

Gay men and women are no different from anyone else except in their sexual orientation. Gradually the prejudices against gay people are being broken down, and in some societies gay couples can now get married and adopt children. South Africa set a very important standard in the world when it refused to discriminate against homosexuals and lesbians in its constitution.

Gender

A person is either male or female, either a man or a woman. The words 'gender' and 'sex' are often used interchangeably, for example when you speak of someone of the opposite gender or sex. Because the word 'sex' has so many possible meanings it is better to use 'gender' when you want to indicate whether someone is male or female. Sex, being the traditional term, is however still used on many official forms and questionnaires where one is asked to state one's gender.

Gender roles are the social functions prescribed by society, e.g. traditionally men are the breadwinners and women are the caregivers; men do construction work and women do the cooking. All gender roles are socially constructed, except for giving birth and suckling an infant (women) and producing sperm* (men) to fertilise the ova. Remember that because these roles are socially constructed they are not written in stone, they can change with the times and as our cultures evolve.

In a school examination paper the question was set: 'Give an account of the creation of man.' A little girl wrote: 'First God created Adam. Then He looked at him and said, "I think, if I tried again I could do better." Then He created Eve.' – Esther Harding

65

Gender discrimination

When someone is treated in a certain way simply because he is a man or she is a woman, they are victims of gender discrimination. According to the South African constitution this is against the law. For example, if a woman is denied a certain job, such as driving a big truck or being a mining engineer, because it is believed that as a woman she will not be able to do that job, she is discriminated against on the grounds of gender.

However, sometimes gender discrimination happens in a way which no constitution can prevent. For example, men are often expected to behave in a certain way because people feel that is the way men have always behaved: men don't cry, because 'cowboys don't cry'. So gender discrimination can be found both in the workplace and in private life, because men and women are often still cast in traditional roles: men are expected to get education*, do the tough jobs and be macho*, while women are expected to look after the house and bring up the children and be subservient and gentle. This is wrong, because if men and women are given equal education and equal opportunities they can perform the same tasks equally well.

Does the law protect you from gender discrimination?
Discrimination on the basis of gender is illegal in South Africa, whether at the hands of the government or a private company or an individual. In Zimbabwe only discrimination by government or a public institution is illegal. Customary law discriminates on the basis of gender in the private sphere, that is within the family or home.

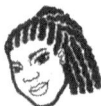

How can I prevent being discriminated against because I am a woman?
The first step is to consider yourself equal to any boy or man. If you believe in your own value as a human being in the first place, and not primarily as a woman, you will act with confidence even if someone tries to belittle you or treats you as inferior or weak because you are a woman.

What is the role of women in traditional societies?
In the past men and women were treated with equal respect* but had clearly defined separate roles. In African society the value placed on women's contribution – to the household and to agricultural labour – was marked by payment of lobola* or bride-price. In Africa, as in many other religions* and cultures, women were regarded as minors (of lesser value and not of full age) and treated as such. A woman needed someone else to represent her or her interests legally, and sometimes she was considered a valuable asset. Traditionally, for example, a family could settle an action for damages, or unite two 'warring' families, by giving their daughter in marriage* to

a member of the other family, even though the daughter might not have wanted to get married to the man. Today this kind of transaction is illegal and a woman can appeal to a court of law should it happen. Arranged marriages do however still occur, and the girl's family is rarely prosecuted for this. In most cases women have the law behind them to enforce gender equality, but most of them lack either the financial resources or the courage to use the power of the law to be considered equal, or to be treated as a major rather than a minor.

Girlfriend

A girlfriend can be described as a boy's or man's usual or favourite companion.

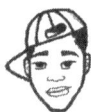

Is it OK for my girlfriend to speak to her friends about our relationship?

A relationship between two people is private and should be treated as such. However, no relationship is absolutely exclusive. Naturally you and your girlfriend will continue to have other friends, and it is not unnatural for her to want to tell one or two close friends of the fun, and the difficulties, you and she are having. Especially if one encounters problems, it is often good to share your worries and seek a second opinion. This does not, however, mean that your girlfriend has the right to gossip about you or your relationship, or to discuss intimate issues behind your back in a way that is not respectful of you or the difficulties you're having.

How should I behave when I meet my girlfriend's parents*?

It is quite natural to be slightly nervous or shy, because it can be an awkward occasion where everyone, even the parents, may feel self-conscious and worry that they might not make a good impression. The best you can do is *not* to try to impress by showing off. Be as natural as possible and keep in mind that you are not the only one feeling this way.

Good-time girl

A 'good-time' girl is a young woman who likes to party and have fun. Some people expect women to be quiet and shy, so they might say she has loose morals. This is because they think women who enjoy socialising and going out also sleep with their social partners. This is not fair, because such a judgement is based on what they assume rather than what they know for a fact, and if a man likes to go out a lot and have fun in the company of women he does not seem to attract the same criticism. Is this just or fair?

Grief

Grief usually arises out of a real loss: losing a person, a place or a way of life. It is natural to feel this way. The important thing is not to push the emotion aside and pretend you are not feeling this way if you are. It is generally easier for girls to cope with grief as society does not criticise them if they cry or mourn*. It is harder for boys who, traditionally, are not supposed to show emotion. However, feelings that are repressed or pushed down often emerge later in life as anger or depression*, sometimes resulting in suicide*.

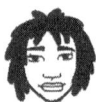

How can I cope with my feelings of grief?

If you are grieving don't feel guilty or ashamed, but allow the emotion to find a release. Talk to someone close to you, and allow yourself to cry. Bear in mind that grief does not go away overnight. Do not push yourself too hard; try to get through one day at a time. Each day try to focus on something that you enjoy doing or which seems worth doing and involve yourself in it totally. Slowly, over time, the feelings of grief will pass.

My best friend is grieving about losing someone she loved very much. What can I tell her?

If someone close to you is grieving, allow her to talk to you. It is often more important to listen than to offer advice. Above all, don't tell her to 'snap out of it' or that someone else has suffered more than she has. Don't deny her the opportunity to express the full impact of the loss she is feeling.

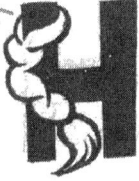

Hangover

The word 'hangover' is used to describe how someone feels when they wake up after having consumed too much alcohol* the previous evening. When you have a hangover you feel groggy and usually have a headache, your mouth is dry and you are thirsty. To cure a hangover drink plenty of cold water. If you think you are going to a party and will drink too much, drink some milk before you go out – this will help to 'line' your stomach. Try to sleep off a hangover rather than taking painkillers.

Heavy petting

Also see Foreplay

Heavy petting is a form of sexual intimacy. It usually involves intense French kissing*, mutual fondling and mutual masturbation*, but does not include actual sexual intercourse*. However, HIV/AIDS* and STIs* may be transmitted by heavy petting.

HIV/AIDS

HIV stands for **H**uman **I**mmunodeficiency **V**irus. HIV is a virus that breaks down or destroys the immune system of humans, which normally fights off infections. You are HIV-positive if the virus is detected in your blood. Over a period of time the virus or the HIV infection will develop through several phases up to a point where the immune system of the body is so severely depleted that it can no longer effectively protect the body against other infection. This phase is referred to as the AIDS phase.

Full-blown AIDS is a disease that once contracted will result in death. The HIV virus is transmitted through body fluids such as blood, semen and vaginal fluids. If the HIV virus has weakened the body's immune system sufficiently any serious infection will cause death. Pneumonia and tuberculosis (TB) are two of the most common AIDS-related causes of death.

How is the HIV virus spread?

The HIV virus is transmitted by contact with body fluids: blood and semen in particular and saliva to a much lesser extent. In order for the virus to spread from one person to another there needs to be an exit point for the virus to leave the body of the infected person and an entry point through which the virus can enter the body of another person. The most common way of contracting the HIV virus is through unprotected sexual intercourse* with an infected partner. The virus can also be contracted through blood transfusions. The other way in which the virus can be contracted is by using infected injection needles – needles that have already been used by infected persons. For this reason drug addicts are very vulnerable and, obviously, also people who have unprotected sex (without a condom*) with many different partners.

The Ugandan
ABC and D of HIV:

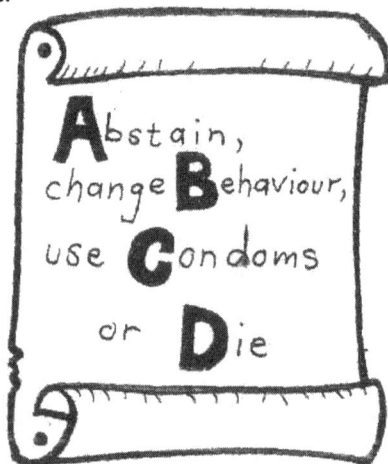

Abstain, change Behaviour, use Condoms or Die

Is there a cure for AIDS?
No. There is presently no known medical cure for AIDS, and no guaranteed way to remove HIV from your body. So-called anti-retroviral drugs, which are very expensive, can help to keep the HIV virus from developing into full-blown AIDS and keep an AIDS sufferer alive and relatively strong and healthy for quite a number of years. In addition, infected people can boost their immune systems by following a proper nutritional diet* and taking care not expose themselves to common viruses that may affect their immune systems, such as the common cold. They may also need additional vitamin supplements to boost their immune systems.

Doesn't sleeping with a virgin cure AIDS?
No! Not even medical science has developed a cure for AIDS yet. It is silly to think that sleeping with a virgin can cure any kind of sickness, let alone an incurable disease such as AIDS. The only thing that will happen if an AIDS-sufferer sleeps with a virgin is that she too will very likely contract the disease.

What does it mean to be HIV-positive?

It means that you have contracted the HIV virus but that it has not yet developed into full-blown AIDS. It is easier to contain the virus at this stage, and identified early enough and properly treated the virus need not develop into AIDS. At this early stage it is very important to lead a healthy lifestyle, eat healthy foods, sleep well and exercise regularly. This way your immune system remains strong and you can delay the onset of full-blown AIDS by many years.

Does this mean that if you are HIV-positive and take care of yourself you won't need anti-retrovirals?

If you have been diagnosed with AIDS, taking good care of yourself will not be enough. You would need anti-retroviral treatment. Anti-retrovirals is a general term for different forms of medication that can help to prevent the onset of AIDS, or at a later stage to keep it under control. These drugs, however, are expensive and few people can afford them, so ideally anti-retrovirals should be provided free of charge. Governments can rarely afford to do so. Recently the South African government initiated a plan to look at the feasibility of providing anti-retrovirals as widely as possible to people who have been diagnosed with AIDS.

When my partner wants to have unprotected sex what should I do?

You have the right – and the responsibility – to protect yourself! Not only can unprotected or unsafe sex lead to pregnancy*, but it is also the most common way in which STIs*, including HIV/AIDS, are transmitted. In fact in South Africa and in Zimbabwe it is a crime to have unprotected sex with someone if you know you are HIV-positive unless you tell that person you are infected and they agree to have unprotected sex. This also applies to husbands or wives. It however remains the responsibility of you as an individual to protect yourself. So unless you know for a fact that your partner is not HIV-positive (and only a medical blood test can tell), and unless he sleeps only with you, you should always insist that he uses a condom*, no matter how unwilling he may be to do so.

My sister, who is very religious, is getting married soon; I know her fiancé has had other girlfriends*, and I am afraid that she might get AIDS.

Both your sister and her boyfriend* should go for an HIV test together before having sex. After the test they should abstain from unprotected sex for three months and then go for another test. This window period is necessary because it can take up to three months before HIV infection can be detected. If the second test is negative it is safe for them to have unprotected sex. But if there is the slightest doubt they should use a condom. Sexual rights come with responsibility: responsibility for yourself and your partner.

How widespread is HIV/AIDS?

According to UNAIDS/WHO 42 million people in the world were living with HIV/AIDS in December 2002; 5 million were infected with HIV during 2002, while 3,1 million died of AIDS-related diseases. Africa south of the Sahara is the worst-affected region. Here 29,8 million people live with HIV/AIDS. Of this number 10 million are young people (aged 15 to 24) and almost 3 million children under 15 are HIV-positive.

In February 2001 the following rates of infection per country in southern Africa were reported: Botswana – 36%; Namibia – 19,5%; Swaziland – 25%; South Africa – 20% and Zimbabwe – 25%. This means one in every five South Africans is infected.

In October 2001 a South African Medical Research Council report said that one person gets infected every minute in South Africa, which means that there are 1 600 new infections per day, with the highest infection rate in the age group 15 to 19 years.

Can I contract AIDS by putting an infected penis* in my mouth?

If the person ejaculates* semen into your mouth there is a strong probability that you may contract the HIV virus. The lining of the inner cheek in your mouth is very sensitive and often has little tears or wounds in the skin. A disease of the mouth, such as bleeding gums can even cause open sores in the mouth. This can be an entry point for the virus. The infected penis is an exit point for the virus, so it is certainly possible to get infected if the man has an orgasm*.

My uncle has AIDS. Will I contract it too?

No. There is no reason why you should contract it from your uncle. The virus is transmitted through body fluids by way of unprotected sexual intercourse*, unscreened blood transfusions or the use of infected injection needles. So, as long as you do not have a blood transfusion using your uncle's blood, you cannot contract the virus from him. And in any case this is unlikely, because these days all blood donors are screened for the HIV virus before they are allowed to donate their blood.

A PERSON WILL NOT BECOME INFECTED WITH HIV THROUGH

pets and insects, such as ticks or mosquitoes

someone else's coughing and sneezing

a handshake, hugging or touching an infected person

sharing the same food, cutlery, toilet seat or shower

swimming in the same swimming pool or

living and working together with an HIV-positive person

What do you do if you discover you are HIV-positive?
Discovering that you are HIV-positive can come as a terrible shock. To help yourself over this difficult period it is best to seek advice from one of the many HIV/AIDS support organisations.

Find out as much as possible about the disease and how you can survive it. It is possible to help keep the virus under control by eating the right foods, not drinking alcohol*, taking exercise and sleeping enough and properly, but you need to be properly informed because a lot of misinformation is spread. So get professional advice.

It is also very important to make sure that you don't infect anyone else through unprotected sex. If you are not already using a condom*, start immediately.

Give yourself time to think about whether you want to tell other people about your status or not. Consider questions such as: What will I gain from telling them? How do I expect them to react? Obviously if you are in a sexual relationship you should tell your partner about your HIV status. This is not an easy thing to do and it takes courage. Your relationship may go through a very difficult period of anger, recrimination, shame, blame, misery, bitterness, even break up – which is another reason why it is important to seek counselling, advice and support for you and your partner. Yet it is essential for an infected person to tell his or her partner, so they too can take the necessary precautions to combat the disease for themselves, and make sure that they do not unknowingly spread it.

Remember that you can be prosecuted if you infected someone while you were aware that you were infected.

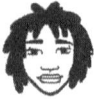

How do I tell my girlfriend* that I'm HIV-positive?

This is not an easy thing to have to do. However, if you have been having sexual relations with your girlfriend you have a strong moral responsibility to inform her as soon as possible. It is important and urgent, because her life could be in danger and she needs to seek medical attention as soon as possible. If you love* and care about her you will tell her, no matter how difficult it is.

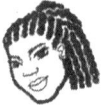

Why does society so often neglect people living with AIDS?

This is mainly out of fear and ignorance. People don't always understand how the virus is spread and they fear that they may contract it simply by social contact with an infected person. Sometimes there is also the stigma attached to people with HIV – it's seen as a curse from God for being sinful, playing around, etc., even when this is obviously untrue. Because of this, society tends to exclude and neglect AIDS sufferers at a time when they need care and attention most. The fact that there is no known cure for the virus as yet makes the fear greater.

Is it OK to seek revenge when someone with HIV/AIDS has slept with you?

No. Treat other people the way you want to be treated. There is a moral and legal obligation on people not to wilfully spread the virus, and to inform their sexual partners of their HIV-positive status if they know it.

In South Africa and in Zimbabwe it is a crime to have unprotected sex with someone if you know you are HIV-positive, unless you tell that person you are infected and he or she agrees to have unprotected sex.

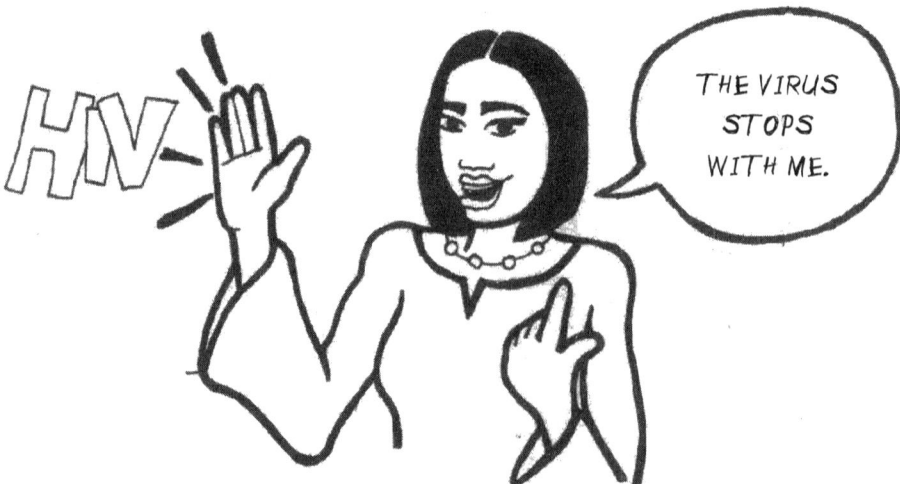

Can I trust someone to tell the truth if he says he is HIV-negative?
It would depend on how well you know the person. To sleep with someone whom you hardly know is to take a huge risk, never mind what he tells you about his status. Better to protect yourself at all times by insisting on safe sex* – on him using a condom. In the end it is the responsibility of each person to protect her- or himself from the virus. Never assume that someone will tell you he or she is HIV-positive. Many people lack the courage to do so. Also remember that many people do not know their HIV status.

Holding hands

Holding hands is one way of showing affection, especially in African society. Friends sometimes hold hands, as well as lovers, siblings, parents and children. Holding hands is safe, warm, feel-good physical contact with a person that you like and trust. But make sure that the other person also likes holding hands, because in some cultures physical contact is not considered a natural way of showing affection, and some people don't like it as much as others.

Homosexuality

Also see Gay

Homosexuality is when a person is physically attracted to another person of the same sex rather than the opposite sex. So the term refers to this type of sexual orientation and to sexual relationships between two men or two women. In everyday language men who are homosexual are often called 'gay'; female homosexuals are sometimes called 'gay' and sometimes called 'lesbians'. A person who is attracted to someone of the opposite gender is called a 'heterosexual'.

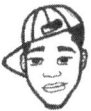

Is there a cure for homosexuality?
No, there isn't a cure, because homosexuality is *not* a disease or an illness. It is one way of expressing your sexuality or sexual orientation. Homosexuals do not choose their sexual orientation – it is something they realise about themselves as they grow into puberty and adolescence, and this realisation may be very difficult and traumatic for them, especially as society is still often prejudiced against them. Gays can't change to suit society, just as heterosexuals can't suddenly become gay.

If you have homosexual feelings, in other words if you feel a sexual attraction to a person of the same gender as yourself, and you are confused or feel it is wrong to have such feelings, or you feel ashamed and worried about what your friends or family will say, you should try to speak to a counsellor who can give you advice and support.

Do gay people have any rights in a court of law?
In South Africa it is illegal to discriminate against somebody on grounds of her or his sexual orientation or preference. Discrimination against homosexuals is therefore illegal and it is legal to have a sexual relationship with a person of the same biological sex. One cannot, however, get married to a person of the same sex. In Zimbabwe it is illegal for gay men to have sexual intercourse* (anal sex*) but it is not illegal for lesbian women to have sexual relations, only because the offence is impossible to prove. However, lesbian women still suffer discrimination because their sexuality is not recognised by society and women are often pressured into marriage* and to bear children.

What does 'coming out' mean?
When a gay or lesbian person tells other people about his or her sexual preference and decides to live openly as a homosexual, it is called 'coming out' or 'coming out of the closet'. In the past, religious institutions and societies all over the world have often had very negative attitudes towards homosexuality. Therefore many gay people kept their desires and feelings secret.

In today's society, people are freer to 'come out' with their true sexual orientation because it has generally become more acceptable. But even so, it is still hard for many gay people to take this step because of lingering social prejudice, which may also affect their family members.

Ultimately, if you want to grow up to be happy and healthy you need to accept your sexual feelings (unless they are harmful to others!) regardless of what other people think. It is often most difficult for gay people to tell their families about their sexual orientation. In such cases they should consider getting counselling to help them work through their feelings about the matter.

Coming out is usually a process that takes time. First it means accepting yourself as gay or lesbian, then telling a friend or your family. It is always better first to tell people who will give you support. And, finally, go public, the stage when it no longer matters to you who knows if you are gay or lesbian. In many societies today there are groups and organisations that stand up for the rights of gay people and try to educate society so that no one will discriminate against them. In every society approximately 10% of the population is gay.

How does society judge homosexuality?

Today most people agree that sexual orientation (whether you are homosexual or heterosexual) is neither normal nor abnormal, except in so far as the majority of people are heterosexual and only up to about 10% of people homosexual. It is a way of being, of expressing your sexuality. Some people feel proud to be homosexual, while others feel ashamed and try to hide it because of traditional or conservative attitudes to homosexuality. In South Africa one finds many different reactions to homosexuality. In the cities few people take any notice of whether you like men or women, and it's OK to be openly homosexual. But in small towns or rural areas there may still be strong disapproval of homosexuality which can even be physically threatening.

In short, some cultures accept homosexuality, others not. Similarly, some families accept homosexuality more easily than others. Sometimes when people who used to be very negative about gays are told their son or daughter is gay they become more open-minded and accepting and more aware of the prejudices against homosexuality.

What is 'homophobia'?

The word means 'an intense and unreasoning hatred of homosexuality and homosexuals' – a form of social hate reflected by a society, or more usually a social group within a society, which intensely dislikes people that are 'different'. They feel threatened by them and want to stamp out what they consider 'deviant' – behaviour that differs from what they think is normal. Homophobia is alive and well among some people in southern Africa. Homosexuals are often a target, and this can lead to violent acts or words directed against them.

However, the South African constitution states that all people should be treated alike and cannot be discriminated against on the grounds of their sexual orientation, so if a gay person is verbally or physically attacked he or she can take the matter to court. In Zimbabwe this does not apply.

How do lesbian women live?

Some women live heterosexual lives, in other words they live with a person of the opposite sex but they also have sexual relations with women. (A person who feels attracted to both men and women is called 'bisexual', 'bi-' meaning 'two' or 'double'.) Other lesbians or gay women make their sexual preference a life choice and are not interested in having men as partners at all. They find a woman whom they love* and the couple become life partners, just like a man and woman who decide to get married.

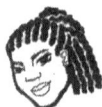

Does fancying your best girlfriend for a while mean you are gay?
No. Many teenagers go through a period of being attracted to people or particular members of the same sex – like having a crush on your same-sex teacher – but later find they are more attracted to people of the opposite sex.

Hormones

There are two types of glands in the body: endocrine glands, which produce hormones, and exocrine glands, which produce digestive juices. The genital glands – the testes* in the man and the ovaries* in the woman – are also part of the endocrine glandular system. As we grow from a small child to a teenager to an adult and eventually into an old person, our bodies keep changing. This is because the endocrine system produces hormones that affect one's body in very specific ways at different stages of one's life: teenagers' skin suddenly becomes oily and spotty; girls develop breasts and wider hips; both boys and girls grow hair around their private parts (genitals)* and boys' voices become deeper. Women start to ovulate (release eggs during a fertile period each month) and menstruate (see menstruation*).

Not just the body, but also the behaviour and mood of human beings are influenced by hormonal changes and processes.

Hugging

Hugging is a great way of giving and receiving warmth and affection. Hugs do not have to be sexual – any two people can hug and it can be a safe, comforting and supportive gesture. There's nothing wrong with asking for a hug from someone you know and care for. Just be sure that the other person too is comfortable with getting and giving a hug.

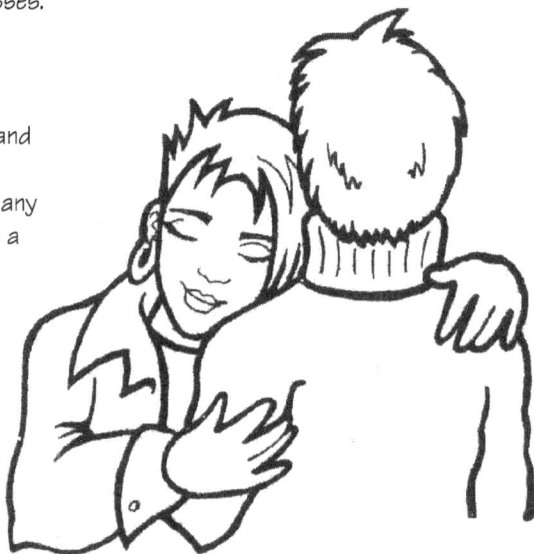

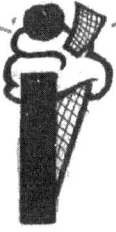

Impotence

Impotence usually means that a man is unable to have an erection or to sustain one. However, the term may also be used when a man is unable to ejaculate, or if he comes too quickly. Reaching a sexual climax too quickly is also called premature ejaculation*. Most men experience all these reactions at some stage or another. Alcohol* and anxiety can make these conditions worse.

Many men find it very difficult to admit that they might have a problem. When it concerns sexual problems women are often more willing to seek advice and treatment.

Incest

Incest is sexual intercourse* within the immediate family. This can include abuse* by an adult in a parental role, e.g. a stepmother or stepfather, or an uncle or an aunt. Incest is punishable by law in South Africa and in Zimbabwe. An adult committing incest can be sent to prison for a long time. Sometime incest takes place because a young girl may be physically and socially unable to defend herself against the sexual actions of a father, uncle or older brother who has the advantage of greater strength and authority over her.

Incest is a social taboo* within most cultures, although different cultures have different ideas on what constitutes incest. For instance in southern Africa there are traditional laws against marriage* between people with the same totem or protective family symbol. Some cultures accept marriage between cousins, while it is strictly forbidden in others.

Incest is a crime even if both the partners are adults and consent to have sexual intercourse. Such incidents are still punishable by law and the offenders may receive a fine or a prison sentence, because if a baby is born as the result of incest the child may have serious mental or physical problems.

When people of the same family produce children it is called 'in-breeding'. Constant in-breeding (as with the Vadema in the north of Zimbabwe) can lead to genetic 'faults' being passed down to the next generation, because people from the same bloodline will have a tendency towards certain diseases.

Infertility is a condition where a man or a woman is unable to have children. This may have a physical cause, e.g. the man may not be able to produce enough sperm*, or it may be psychological, e.g. if the woman is too anxious or inhibited. For this reason it is not unusual that a woman falls pregnant after she and her husband have adopted a child. In other words, having a child reduces the tension about being able to have a child.

Men and women are very often treated differently if they are infertile. Infertility is often blamed on the woman and may be cited as a reason for divorce* or desertion. If the man is infertile, some African societies allow his wife to have sex with his brother in a very private way so that she can fall pregnant and produce a baby to save the family honour. If the woman turns out to be infertile, she is often sent back to her parents*. Modern African societies do not encourage this practise due to the HIV/AIDS* pandemic.

Today, as more couples decide not to have children, the stigma attached to being childless has diminished. There are also numerous fertility treatments available for couples who are experiencing problems having children.

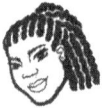

I have heard that STIs* can make you infertile. Is that true?

Yes, in some cases. For conception to occur, a live sperm from a man has to 'meet' and fuse with an ovum (egg)* from a woman. This meeting happens in the woman's Fallopian tubes*. When STIs like gonorrhoea go untreated they may infect the woman's sexual organs and cause swelling and inflammation that in turn could cause blockage of the tubes, leading to infertility. In men, STIs may cause inflammation and subsequent blockage of the ducts. Because of these problems, infertility can occur as the result of STIs.

Is a man with only one testicle infertile?

A man with one testicle* should be perfectly fertile. The testicles produce the sperm required to fertilise the egg. With one testicle a man will produce half the normal amount of sperm, but this should still be more than enough to ensure the fertilisation of one egg.

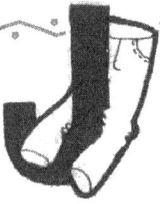

Jealousy

Jealousy is feeling resentment or envy on account of known or suspected or imagined rivalry between you and another person or persons. A jealous person often feels possessive of his partner, believing that he or she should not give any attention to anybody else. This is because he or she feels threatened.

Why do I feel so jealous when my girlfriend* speaks to other guys?
Think very carefully about the matter. Are you perhaps feeling insecure because your girlfriend is not giving you enough attention? Do you feel insecure because you do not know if she really loves you? Is she flirting* with these guys or just having a normal conversation? Try to discuss your feelings with her when the two of you are alone and you are not feeling jealous. Don't get worked up and don't accuse her, discuss it calmly. If she is not giving you any reason to be jealous, you must question your own insecurity and try to fight it.

I was unfaithful to my girlfriend only once. I told her and said I'm sorry. Why does she still act so jealous?
You must understand that your girlfriend feels threatened, so you need to be patient and build up her trust in you again. If you show that you mean what you say, she will regain her confidence in you over time. If it doesn't happen and she can't forget the past, it might be better if you agree to move on – but try not to make the same mistake again! If someone is important to you, be loyal and faithful*.

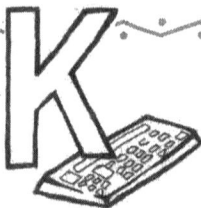

Kissing

To kiss is to touch someone with your lips as a sign of love*, affection, greeting or reverence. One can kiss someone on many places, but usually it is on the mouth, the cheek, the forehead or the hand. You can also blow a kiss to someone, and if you really adore someone people might say: 'He or she kisses the ground on which So-and-so walks.'

Can you greet someone with a kiss?

In many cultures both kissing and hugging* are taboo* in public. However, in as many cultures friends and acquaintances kiss each other when they meet: the English press a kiss on one cheek, the French kiss on both cheeks, the Dutch kiss three times on the two cheeks and the Afrikaners kiss on the mouth. All these cultures shake hands if it is a formal meeting. So whether you kiss when you meet would depend on your culture and how well you know the other person. Generally men do not kiss other men, except in Latin cultures where it is not uncommon, though in many cultures they hug each other. You should only kiss someone if it feels right to you. Of course when friends or family kiss you it is very different from the way lovers kiss each other.

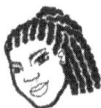

How do lovers kiss?

Kissing between two people who love each other is an intimate act and one not usually seen in public, except in the movies! Lovers usually open their mouths when they kiss, allowing their tongues to touch (see French kissing*). It is sometimes called 'wet kissing'.

Is it healthy to kiss?

A lovers' kiss can't be very healthy at the best of times, but some infections are specifically spread through this kind of wet kissing. Glandular fever, for example, can be spread through saliva (spit). Herpes, a common STI*, can also be contracted through kissing and contact with the fluid in the cold-sore blister in the corner of the affected person's mouth. Even the HIV* virus can be spread through wet kissing.

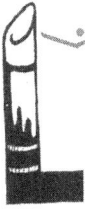

Lesbians see Gay, Homosexuality

Lobola

Lobola or bride-price* is an ancient African custom whereby money or goods are handed to a bride's family by the groom's family to indicate that the families agree to a marriage*. The bride's family sets the price. Traditionally cattle were given, but today the price is often set in terms of money. Lobola has different functions in different ethnic groups, but generally it is a token of the union of the two families and shows that the groom's family is gaining a woman who will bear children and provide labour for them. Lobola is not a requirement to make a customary-law marriage binding, but may be proof that such a union exists. Lobola may include 'penalties' – an extra amount of money or goods if the woman and the man have had a sexual relationship prior to the lobola ceremony. The price will also increase if the woman has had a child.

Love

There are many different forms and definitions of love. The love for one's parents*, siblings, children, or friends is different from love you feel for your boyfriend*/girlfriend*, lover, or husband/wife. A sexual relationship based on love always involves faithfulness* and commitment*. Such a relationship normally starts with 'falling in love' – a magical experience characterised by intense emotions. Usually this is just a passing phase. Lasting love between partners is a complex emotion that develops and changes over time, as the two partners get to know and appreciate each other more and more. Mutual respect* and consideration are essential in this kind of enduring love.

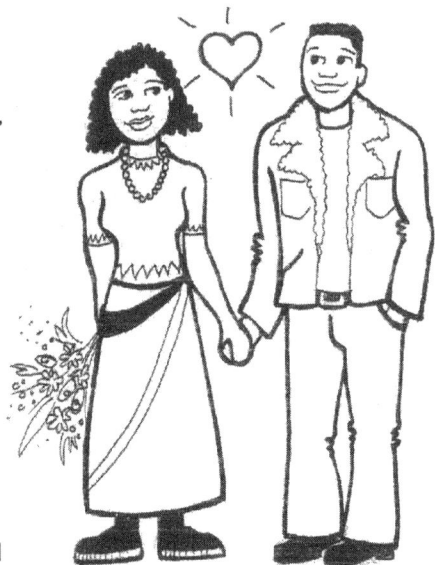

Love is a fan club with only two fans!

How do I know that I am in love?

When people fall in love they are drawn together by a powerful attraction*. Sometimes it is simply physical lust, at other times the attraction is a mixture being drawn together by each other's personality and physical presence.

You know you are 'in love' when you are infatuated with someone and can't stop thinking about him, when you daydream about him, remember every word he said to you, the way he looked at you. You may or may not have erotic thoughts about him, but you will certainly feel excited when you are near him. These are the signs of being in love. If the infatuation grows into a deeper emotion of love, the sensation of intense excitement will disappear and your feelings will develop into an understanding and acceptance of the other person.

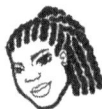

Does 'true love' exist?

True love does exist, but it is not like movie romances or love stories make us believe. True love is about honesty, friendship*, loyalty, mutual support and respect*. Lasting true love does not happen overnight. It takes time for real love to grow, because it is a deep emotional connection to the other person, involving trust, faithfulness* and commitment*. One good definition of true love is 'caring more about what happens to the loved one than about what happens to yourself'.

A meaningful relationship grows with time, and often has its ups and downs, so a couple must be prepared to work at the relationship, resolving emotional and other problems together.

Will I fall in love only once in my life?

Probably not. Most people fall in love several times in the course of their lives. Having a first boyfriend* or girlfriend* is like a staging post in the process. You think you'll love someone for ever and ever, but especially if you are young something can happen that causes you to break up. You might get hurt, but it is not the end of the world. In the process you get to know your own strengths and weaknesses and you come out of the unhappiness more grown-up, and you move on.

The important thing is that if and when you finally decide to get married you fully understand the implications of the decision; that you are completely sure and mature enough then to be prepared to share your life with the other person for ever, 'come rain or shine', as the saying goes.

Falling in love with someone else when you are married usually causes a lot of upheaval and unhappiness. It can be much more destructive and hurtful than any previous experience of falling in love you have had, because now not only two people are affected. Especially if there are children, it can lead to more trauma than happiness.

Is love at first sight possible?

Yes, if your intuition, as well as the other person's, is very good. Some couples can vividly remember the first time they met and boast that it was 'love at first sight'. However, realistically speaking, two people need to get to know each other before they can be sure they love each other. Love at first sight is based on a flash of attraction and can be very superficial. In some cases it can turn into true love, if your intuitions are correct, but more often the relationship breaks up because both people turn out to be very different from the first impression they formed of each other.

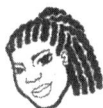

What should I do if a guy tells me he loves me?

It depends on whether you love him too. If you don't, but you believe that he is sincere about his feelings, you should be polite and caring so that he is not hurt. Tell him that you like him for whatever his qualities are, but that you don't love him. Don't pretend something you don't feel.

If you feel that he only says he loves you because he wants to get you into bed, treat it lightly or change the topic. Don't feel pressured to return the compliment if you don't like him.

If you love the person in the same way he says he loves you, you will know exactly what to do!

What should I do if I am too shy to tell a guy that I love him?

There are other ways of expressing your feelings than saying it in words. For instance, writing a letter might be easier than telling him to his face. You can also ask someone else to let him know how much you care. However, getting the message to him in such an indirect way can lead to misunderstandings – imagine how hurt you would be if a message came back to you that he does not feel the same way.

It is always better to observe someone's body language when you tell him something important – the expression on his face, whether he moves closer to you, that kind of thing. So it is probably best to pluck up courage and tell him yourself how you feel. These days it is not necessary any more to wait for the boy to approach you first. Women are in any case much better at expressing themselves than men are!

What should I do if I fall in love with a guy and he doesn't notice?
This is a common dilemma and it is one of the hard parts about being a teenager. Sometimes a girl that likes a guy without him noticing is happy to daydream about him until her intense feelings finally pass. On the other hand, she may long to tell him about her feelings. By doing so she is however taking a risk, because she doesn't know what his response will be. Nobody else can decide for her if she should take the chance or not.

It's important to have good friends with whom you can share your feelings, hopes and wishes. Talking about these things helps to put them in perspective. Besides friends, it is also good to have hobbies and other interests, so that if the guy doesn't like you as much as you like him you can amuse yourself in another way.

Whatever the guy's response, remember your life and your self-esteem do not depend on him loving you too. You are your own person and it would be nice if he liked you too, but it is not a catastrophe if he doesn't. There are many other monkeys in the forest!

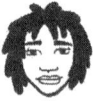

What is the difference between love and sex?
Love is a deep feeling of commitment*, caring and devotion: wanting to share your life with someone. Ideally, one's lover should be one's best friend too. Lovers should be able to talk and laugh together, have the same or similar values, enjoy each other's differences but share similar interests. When you really love someone, and want to hold her or kiss her, a sexual relationship with her will follow naturally.

Sex is a physical urge that demands satisfaction. So some people can enjoy having sex with someone they hardly know and don't love. In the long run this does not satisfy them however. Most people ultimately do not enjoy intimate physical contact with someone they don't love.

What should I do if a guy asks me to show him my private parts?
Tell him to:

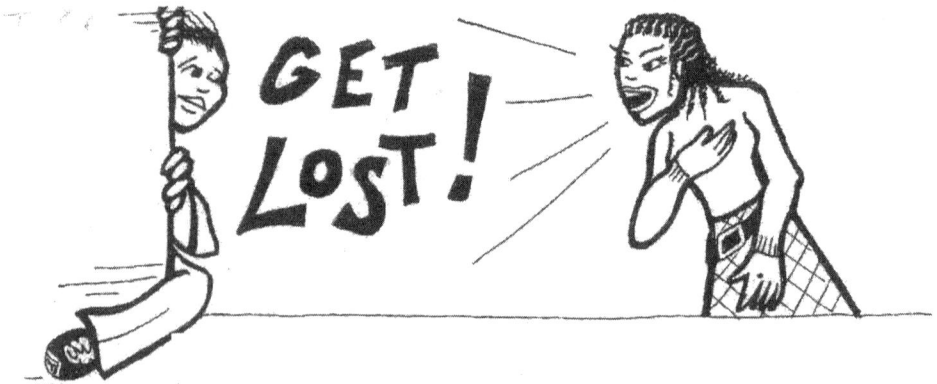

GET LOST!

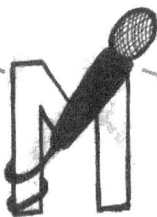

Macho

To be called 'macho' is not a compliment, because the word describes men who think more about their bodies, their image and their sexual prowess and virility than anything else. Macho men often feel they have to maintain an image of being tough and rough. Macho and 'masculine' are not the same. Masculine means 'manly' – like a man.

Why do some guys act macho?
Macho men are often afraid that if they don't act tough they will be accused of being weak, or even of having been bewitched by a woman. Often macho men are actually quite insecure under their façade of toughness, and only boast of their strength or superiority to cover their feelings of inadequacy. A man who is sure of himself doesn't need to show off.

Manners

Also see Courtesy

To have manners is to know how to behave in a social environment. Because children are taught manners at home, people say someone with good manners has 'good breeding'. Manners is not very different from 'etiquette', which is 'the conventional rules of personal behaviour in polite society'. Often good manners are the way we show consideration for the feelings of others. People with good manners treat poor or helpless people with the basic respect* they would show to the rich and powerful – or their own family.

What is the difference between good manners and bad manners?
Every culture, society and class has different ideas about what constitutes good manners. In Victorian England, for example, people's behaviour and manners were governed by very strict rules. Things have changed very much since then. Most people live in multi-cultural societies now, so there are not so many hard and fast rules about manners any more. However, most people still appreciate others who are polite and considerate, and polite and considerate people almost automatically display good manners. Basic good manners means offering respect to people who are older than

you, being courteous and welcoming to strangers, and not putting your-self first. To mention a few concrete examples:

* Do not push through a door first, but stand aside for others;
* Offer your seat on the bus or train to an older person without a seat;
* Explain the way to a stranger who is obviously lost;
* Do not call someone older than you by their first name when they have not given you permission to do so.

Another guideline for good manners is not to behave in a way that would make other people uncomfortable:

* Do not eat with your mouth open;
* Do not talk with your mouth full of food;
* Do not spit when you talk;
* Do not dig in your nose with your finger;
* Do not scratch your armpit;
* Do not talk at the same time as someone else;
* Do not talk loudly in a public place where other people too are having conversations;
* Do not rush to use the telephone or toilet in someone else's house without asking permission first.

In short, people with good manners are pleasant to have around you, while people without manners are a pain in the neck.

Why do teenagers often display bad manners when they are away from their parents*?

Probably because they are more insecure than mature, and because they are trying to assert their independence. They do not realise that they are creating a bad impression, because they are too self-centred.

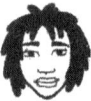

What constitutes good table manners?

These will vary from culture to culture and household to household, but very basic general rules are:

* Do not tuck into your food until everyone has been served;
* Look around the table to see if you need to pass anything to anyone;
* Remember to thank your hostess afterwards;
* Do not rush away from the table until everyone has finished eating.

Whether you eat with your hands or use a knife and fork, and how you use a knife and fork, would depend on your culture. The way you drink your tea, or eat spaghetti, or roast chicken, or porridge (pap/sadza) will depend on your culture and where you were brought up.

Marriage is the legal act of committing yourself to another person for life, in a traditional arrangement, civil or community court, or in a church. There are different forms of marriage contracts and a couple needs to consider all options before they make a choice of contract. It is worthwhile getting legal advice before you sign a marriage contract, from an attorney or from Legal Aid.

Why do people get married?

People marry for different reasons. Some couples say they got married for love*, but one of the most important reasons is that marriage ensures that after the death of one partner the remaining partner has a legal right to the estate (the property) of the deceased spouse. Thus a marriage contract creates security for children born from the marriage and offers financial security for the surviving partner.

Also, because the public administration systems are based on family units, tax laws, medical aid and pension schemes, housing subsidies, child support and many other systems favour married couples above single people. So marriage often has financial benefits in everyday life.

However, these benefits are not enough to make two people marry who do not want to live together. In the end people marry because they want to share their lives and possessions.

Why do some people say marriage is outdated?

They say that because society and the roles of men and women have changed so drastically over the last century. Before, the man used to be the sole breadwinner and the woman stayed home to clean the house and prepare food and bring up the children. Unmarried women were often social outcasts.

But this has all changed and many women are now well educated and have highly paid jobs. Women having to fulfil two roles, some people argue that marriage puts them in an unfair position and robs them of their rights. However, even in some Christian marriage vows women no longer have to promise to 'obey' their husbands. So their equality is also recognised by the church.

The good thing is that all these changes have made it possible for a woman to make a real choice. It is no longer necessary for her to marry for financial security or social standing. If she chooses to marry today it is because wants to make a public commitment* to her husband so that other people can acknowledge the relationship.

What is an arranged marriage and is it recognised by the law?

It is a marriage organised by the parents*, guardians or the families of one or both marriage partners. For any marriage to be legal and binding both partners must consent to the marriage. So if someone is forced into an arranged marriage she can refuse to consent and the arrangement will have to be cancelled. This does not often happen though, either because the woman doesn't know that she has this right or she does not want to disobey her parents or guardians.

Often, but not always, neither the man nor the woman getting married has much say over the choice of partner and the arrangement. Marriages are usually arranged for financial, political, social or religious reasons, to bind two families together. In cultures where arranged marriages are the norm, parents say that because they love their children and know them well they are in the best position to decide whom they should marry.

It is a fact that if both partners in an arranged marriage agree to make it a success and work at their relationship they often end up being happy and loving each other. However, the majority of young people find arranged marriages old-fashioned and feel they should choose their own life partner and 'marry for love'.

Perhaps young people are now more critical or choosy. They believe they can be more selective than in the past because they have more choice – societies are generally more open, and it is much easier for people to meet others of a different culture or class.

Do forced marriages still take place today?

Yes, but not as often as in the past, because the law does not permit it, more particularly if the child is a minor (under the legal age of adulthood, which is 18). Girls are however still forced into marriage by parents who wish to hide 'the shame' of a pregnancy*, or to negotiate financial gain from an unplanned pregnancy. Parents might also promise their daughter to an older man in return for payment, in the form of food or money. Traditionally in African culture a sister or female relative of a deceased wife may be required (forced) to take her place by marrying the widower.

If a young woman is being pressured or forced into marriage for whatever reason she should seek help from a local youth or support group, such as Childline*.

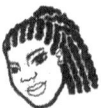

Is it right for a young girl to marry an older man?

People are often critical when an older man marries a much younger woman, because they generally expect that people of more or less the same age should marry. They question the motive behind the marriage, thinking that the girl probably just wants his money or that the man just wants her young body. This is usually just speculation and there is no real reason why such a relationship should not work. An older man may in fact be kinder, gentler, less demanding and more thoughtful than a younger man; a younger girl may be looking for security, and may bring a freshness and joy that an older woman might have lost.

There is an ancient saying that goes: 'Rather an old man's darling than a young man's slave'!

However, a young girl should never be forced into marriage with an older man. This would be wrong.

What is meant by a married woman becoming an inheritance?

In traditional African society if a wife dies a younger sister or a female relative may be required to take her place in the marriage. If the husband dies, the widow is considered to be the property of her husband's male relations and can become the property of her husband's oldest living brother. So in a way her husband's older brother inherits her. Traditionally this was seen as a way of ensuring that the widow and her children were properly looked after. Today, however, a woman who consents to being thus 'inherited' may lose all her matrimonial property.

This practice holds another danger as well because of the threat of HIV/ AIDS* and it has in fact led to the spread of HIV within families.

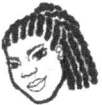

How can a married woman protect herself from contracting HIV?

There is only one way: by ensuring that her husband uses a condom*. If she is not 100% sure that her husband is faithful* to her she should insist that he uses a condom – unless she is planning to have a baby. If she is not sure of her husband's HIV status and condoms are not an option, she should insist on an HIV test before she takes the risk.

This might be very difficult though for women in traditional African marriages. They often have very little, if any, control or say over how many children they will bear, as they are not allowed to practise birth control*. Nor can they insist that their husband uses a condom, even if he has other women. Thus they are forced to have unprotected sex, which makes them extremely vulnerable. Recent research has shown that married women in Zimbabwe are at greater risk of becoming infected with HIV than anyone else. This is a truly tragic situation.

What about being married to more than one wife at the same time?

In our region customary law does allow polygamy*. This is an ancient practice from the time when most young men were away from home fighting wars, with many young women but few men left behind. A modern marriage contract is between one man and one woman only.

Why can't I have more than one partner when I'm married?

If you do you will be breaking a promise. Why get married if you want other women besides your wife? Perhaps you should ask yourself the following questions before you start having sex with multiple partners: What would I do if my partner (or wife) behaved in the same way? What is the risk of HIV/AIDS*? Who am I endangering through my behaviour? Is sleeping around really that much fun?

Is it wise to marry when you are young?

It depends on *how* young. Good marriages hinge on the maturity of the couple, their knowledge of themselves, their shared beliefs, values, and hopes for the future. If you are older you are more likely to have fewer unrealistic expectations of your partner and the marriage and will realise that marriage is something you have to work at. Being young is a time to do all the things a married person cannot easily do: get an education*, travel, experiment with clothes and fashion, go dancing and so on. By the time you get married you should have had enough fun to be ready to settle down and commit yourself to working at the relationship.

What is a marriage proposal?

In most cultures it is the man who proposes marriage to the woman and not vice versa. It simply means that he asks her to marry him. Traditionally he must however seek the permission of the girl's father first.

In Western society the couple become formally engaged if the girl accepts. The man buys the girl an engagement ring, which as his fiancée she wears on the fourth finger of her left hand. Even though it is unlikely that a man will propose before he is fairly certain that the girl will say 'yes', she still has the right to say 'no' if she feels she does not love him, or is not ready for marriage, or wants to remain single.

An engagement precedes the wedding*, and in the olden days this period of being formally betrothed to each other allowed the couple to get to know each other better.

Is sex before marriage acceptable?

In many religions* and cultures sex before marriage is unacceptable and children born out of wedlock are considered illegitimate. However, marriage and sex are two distinct concepts. One may be emotionally and physically ready for sex but not for marriage. If you decide to have pre-marital sex and your belief system allows you to do so, take the necessary precautions to prevent pregnancy* and STIs*. If you are a girl, remember that you may see sex with a partner as a form of commitment* to him but that he may not. He may simply consider the experience a conquest.

In some African cultures the man's family need to be assured that their future daughter-in-law can bear children, and so a couple will not formally marry until a child has been born (or is on the way). When societies did not have access to modern medicine and the survival of the family depended on procreation and many children this practice made sense. Today, however, many people feel this attitude suggests that neither the man nor his family have any respect* for the girl as a person, but simply see her as a breeding animal.

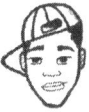

Why can't teenagers get married?

Teenagers can marry if they are over 18 and even earlier, at 16, provided their parents* or guardians consent. But teenage marriage is not a good idea. Good marriages depend on the maturity of the couple and on someone earning a regular income to support the couple and any children they may have. Few teenagers earn enough to set up on their own, so this fact alone places great stress on the young couple. Also, when someone marries very young he or she normally foregoes the opportunity to study further and to lead a carefree life that becomes impossible when you take on the responsibilities of a marriage and a family.

Can there be abstinence* from sex in a marriage?

Yes, for various reasons. Firstly, if you don't want sex for whatever reason – because you are tired, or you no longer enjoy it, or you're afraid to contract a STI, or you don't want to fall pregnant – you should say so. A partner has no right to force you to have sex. Traditionally, women abstained from sex during menstruation*, late pregnancy and breastfeeding and their husbands respected their decision. Today women are increasingly choosing abstinence if they suspect that they may be at risk of HIV infection from their husbands.

Does a married woman have the right to refuse her husband?
Yes and no. Some countries recognise a woman's right to refuse sex within marriage, others, such as Zimbabwe, do not. Rape* within marriage is very difficult to prove, although there are some recorded cases. Men should always pay attention when a woman says 'no' and never insist on having sex with her against her wishes.

Masturbation

Masturbation is when you stimulate your own external genital organs (private parts) to achieve sexual pleasure, usually orgasm*.

Do only men and boys masturbate?
No, some girls and women masturbate too.

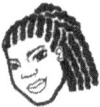

Is masturbation abnormal?
No, it is a healthy release and most people do it. However, when masturbation becomes so important to someone that it becomes an obsession, that person might end up not being able to have sex with a partner. That is obviously a very unhealthy situation.

I've heard that masturbation can make you ill.
There is a myth that masturbation can sap your strength or make you blind. This is not true. Some people say it stems from an ancient belief that it was sinful to waste seed, which was needed to procreate as many children as possible.

Can masturbation break one's virginity*?
No. It is not the same as sexual intercourse*, during which a woman is penetrated.

Why is masturbation associated with feelings of guilt?
Not everybody feels guilty about masturbation, but the guilt normally comes from the way we have been brought up. You may think that your parents* or religion* would disapprove. Masturbation also often involves fantasy, and if you fantasise about someone you shouldn't be dreaming of you may feel your thoughts are impure.

Masturbation is a private activity and it harms no one. If you have strong sexual urges that cannot be fulfilled, masturbation often makes you feel better, even if you feel slightly depressed afterwards.

Menstruation

The 'bleeding' which fertile women experience once a month. Girls begin to menstruate when their bodies begin to develop during adolescence. During a woman's menstrual cycle the wall of the uterus* thickens with blood in readiness to receive the fertilised egg. When this does not happen, the thickening is released over a period of three to seven days as a discharge of blood (menses) and other fragments from the membrane of the uterus. Women who are under stress or suffer from famine or anorexia* will often cease to menstruate.

In some cultures menstruation is celebrated as a sign that the girl has become a woman. Quite often today, if girls are unprepared by their mothers, aunts or older sisters, it can be a little bit frightening for them when they see the blood for the first time.

Menstruation is sometimes accompanied by cramps and the best thing to do is to lie down and take it easy.

What do girls use to absorb the discharge of blood?

Many girls use sanitary pads, which are made of layers of cotton. A sanitary pad is placed between your legs and kept in place by your panties. Other girls use tampons made of compressed cotton, which are placed inside the vagina* and pulled out by means of a piece of cotton string. Both pads and tampons must be changed regularly, because they will stop being effective after they have absorbed a certain amount of blood.

What do I do when I have my period and can't afford pads?

You have a few options on how to make your own if you cannot afford to buy pads:

- Cut or tear a clean old linen or cotton sheet into strips broad enough to fit between your legs. Fold each strip into pads the length and thickness you want. These cloth pads will be soaked quite quickly if your period is heavy, so you need to change the cloth pads and wash yourself frequently to prevent the smell of blood. To keep the pads from soaking right through onto your clothes you can insert a piece of plastic between the outer folds of the cloth. After use these cloth strips must be soaked and washed before you can re-use them.
- If you are fortunate and can get a sheepskin – not goat or cow skin – you can cut the skin into strips the size of a pad or a shape that will fit you. But first you must prepare and knead the skin until it is nice and soft. The clean woolly surface must be worn against your skin. Sheepskin pads are very absorbent and versatile, but you must still change them

regularly to prevent blood leaking onto your clothes. For greater comfort you can sew cloth loops onto each end of the pad and secure them with another strip of cloth around your waist. If sheepskin pads are soaked and washed regularly they can be used and re-used for years.

- If you have neither old cloth nor sheepskin, use paper. Newspaper or brown paper must first be rubbed between your hands until it is soft. Then you fold it into the size and shape that will fit between your legs. Unfortunately paper gets soaked very quickly, so paper pads need to be changed very regularly to prevent giving off an unpleasant smell. It is therefore also extremely important to wash yourself regularly. If you are not a heavy bleeder you can use toilet paper rolled into the shape and size of a pad. Paper pads cannot be re-used.

Is it OK to carry on like normal when I have my period?
When you have your period you are not ill. You might experience cramps, for which painkillers can help. If you feel tired while you have your period just make sure you get more rest than usual, but is not necessary to stay home or in bed – you can even take part in sport. Washing regularly is particularly important during your period.

Molesting

Also see   Abuse, Child abuse, Sexual harassment

Molesting is when anybody touches another person against the other person's wishes. The most common form of molestation is when men force themselves upon women physically. However, very occasionally women also molest men, children or other women. Men also molest other men and boys. Any form of molestation is against the law and is punishable with a fine, or prison sentence if it is serious.

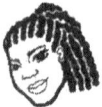

How can one protect oneself from unwanted physical contact?
Try to avoid ever being alone with a boy or man who makes you feel uncomfortable. Shout loudly if there is anyone near enough to hear if you are in a difficult situation.

If you can learn to do a karate chop, all the better, because one chop and any man who is making a nuisance of himself will look at you with renewed respect*. Most bullies are cowards at heart. Nonetheless, violence can feed violence and should only, if ever, be used as a last resort if you feel that you will otherwise be raped* or harmed in some way. Before you counter-attack your molester, make sure you can get away quickly.

Why don't men listen when women say no?
Because they are selfish. If a man disregards your feelings and forces you to do something *he* wants, he is showing no respect* or concern for you. What is more, someone who forces you to have sex with him after you've said 'no' is actually guilty of rape*, which needs to be reported. Be clear in your own mind what you want. Never *pretend* to say 'no', because your partner will sense that you are saying one thing but wanting another. This can cause great problems when you really mean 'no'. Be assertive when you say 'no'.

Morning sickness

Nausea and vomiting that occur during early pregnancy*. In some women the symptoms disappear if a small amount of food is eaten.

Mourning

When someone dies it is usually followed by a period of mourning, during which the bereaved family and friends openly show their grief* about the death of the loved one. People mourn in different ways, depending on their culture and their customs. In most societies mourning is associated with wearing black, either a full outfit or just a ribbon or an armband. There are particular traditional rituals associated with mourning, for example burning the deceased person's clothes or burning candles or incense.

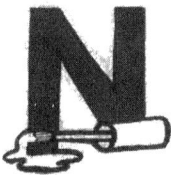

Nutrition

Also see *Diet*

There is no real difference between the terms 'food' and 'nutrition'. Food that is nutritious helps to build and maintain body and mind, and to keep the entire human being integrated, healthy and functional. Nutritious food is rich in vitamins and minerals.

Also see Diet

Obesity

A person who is unhealthily overweight is said to suffer from 'obesity'. An obese person weighs about 30% more than his or her ideal bodyweight. Obesity is a serious risk to health. It is becoming a grave public health problem in many countries and leads to serious chronic diseases, including heart disease and diabetes.

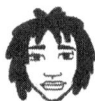

People often tease my girlfriend* that she is fat. Yet she does not eat very much. What is the matter?

Even if she is not eating very much your girlfriend might be taking in more food than her body needs or 'burns off' through exercise. It could also be that her diet* is unhealthy and that she is eating the wrong kinds of food. Certain types of food, especially snacks, are very high in sugars and fats. This could be the reason why she is putting on weight.

However, one's body size is genetic, that is, inherited, which means some people are naturally more plump than others.

On the other hand obesity could be the result of malfunctioning glands, so if your girlfriend doesn't eat sweet things and she exercises regularly she should consult a doctor.

Is dieting the best way to lose weight?

No, not if you mean going on a strict diet to lose weight quickly. Instant diets never work, because if you lose weight quickly you regain it as quickly. In fact, stringent diets that are followed for a long time can be harmful to your health and even lead to anorexia*. The best way to lose weight permanently is to develop a healthy eating pattern and follow a balanced diet – eating lots of fresh vegetables and fruit, cutting out sweet things and fatty foods, eating moderate quantities of carbohydrates (starch) and drinking a maximum of one beer or two glasses of wine per day (because alcohol* too contains lots of sugar). And very important: exercise regularly – take a brisk walk of 20 to 30 minutes at least three times a week. And remember to drink lots and lots of good, clean water – some people say one needs to drink 2 litres of water a day to stay healthy!

One-night stand

A 'one-night stand' is when two people get together to for one night only and share sex without making any other commitment to each other. Such an arrangement can only work if both people want the same thing.

Men sometimes boast about their one-night stands. All it means is that they have no intention of offering affection or commitment*, or sometimes even kindness.

To have a one-night stand if you are craving affection or a steady relationship means that you are likely to get hurt. Remember the risks of contracting STIs* or HIV* are greatly increased by having many partners.

Oral contraception see Contraception

Oral sex

Oral sex is the direct contact between someone's mouth and another's genitals, either as foreplay* or as a way of achieving orgasm*. The oral sex that a woman performs on a man is sometimes called a 'blow job'.

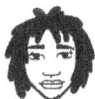

Is there anything wrong with oral sex?
Many people in loving relationships perform oral sex on each other. As with any other sexual activity, it is wrong only if someone is forced to do it against her or his will.

Can I catch HIV/AIDS through oral sex?
Any STI can be spread through oral sex, but not as easily as through genital or anal sex*. You can, however, almost definitely be infected if you have open sores in your mouth or bleeding gums and your partner is HIV-positive and ejaculates in your mouth.

What makes oral sex so enjoyable?
What makes any sex enjoyable?

Oral sex has the advantage of being free from the fear of pregnancy* and certainly carries less risk than sexual intercourse* of transmitting sexually transmitted infections. Enjoyment should, however, be mutual, because on one level one partner is doing all the hard work and the other is receiving all the pleasure! Some people don't like it at all.

Orgasm

An orgasm is a sexual climax. It is also known as 'coming'. It is a highly pleasurable physical sensation which arises in the genitals and then sweeps throughout the whole body. In men it includes ejaculation* of sperm*. In women an orgasm may seem to be less dramatic and less easily determined, but it usually involves some contraction of the vaginal muscles.

How do women achieve an orgasm?
Women and men often require additional stimulation over and above the presence of the penis* in the vagina* to achieve orgasm (see foreplay*). Women usually require stimulation of the clitoris. Since women have different needs in reaching orgasm it is important that men should find out what works best for them.

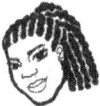

Does one have to have an orgasm when one has sex?
In a sexual relationship it is not always essential for the couple to reach orgasm in order to share intimacy. However, an orgasm releases sexual tension and without that release your partner may feel frustrated.

My lover never makes me climax. Does this mean he doesn't love me?
No, not necessarily. Men are not born with innate knowledge of how women's bodies work, and vice versa – you both have to learn. Your partner may just be inexperienced. Try to tell him what you would like him to do. Some people are too shy to talk about these things, but this can lead to great unhappiness and dissatisfaction. So if you are not comfortable speaking about it, then guide his hand when you are having sex and show him where and how you want him to touch you. If he doesn't respond, it could mean that he is selfish and only thinking of himself.

What does 'frigidity' mean?
In medical terms a frigid woman has difficulty coming to orgasm*. However, few women are truly frigid. Often they simply have had bad experiences with uncaring or inexperienced men in the past, and this has affected their ability to relax and enjoy a loving and caring sexual relationship. The term is often used incorrectly by men to describe a woman who doesn't fancy them and does not want to have sex with them! So if someone tells you you are frigid, ignore him!

A fertile woman's ovaries produce at least one ovum (egg)* per month. The ovum is released into a Fallopian tube* and moves down to the uterus (womb)*, and if it is reached by a sperm* (spermatozoon) on its way there, the ovum will be fertilised and a foetus will begin growing. If more than one ovum is produced during ovulation and fertilised, a woman can become pregnant with twins (or triplets).

Also see the description of the reproductive organs* and the diagram on page 121.

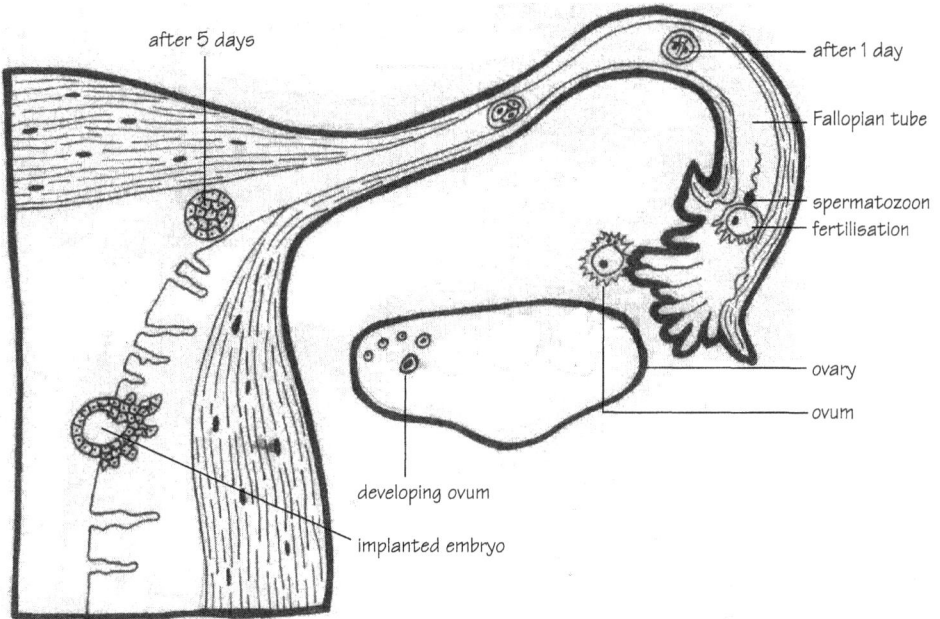

after 5 days

after 1 day

Fallopian tube

spermatozoon
fertilisation

ovary

ovum

developing ovum

implanted embryo

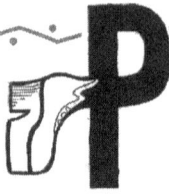

P

Paedophile

A paedophile is a grown-up who takes a sexual interest in children. Some paedophiles become sexually stimulated by looking at pictures of children, but many others force children to perform sexual acts with them. This is punishable by law, and all paedophiles should be reported. Most paedophiles are people with deep-seated psychological and emotional problems who need help desperately, but they will seldom admit that they have a problem.

Parents

Parents are people who have taken the responsibility of producing and raising children. Raising children means taking care of their needs: ensuring they eat enough, have clothes, receive an education* and have a safe place to stay.

To produce a child there are two people involved: a man and a woman – the biological or birth parents. Often children are raised by one parent only (single parent*). When a married couple with children separate they are still parents, and many divorced parents share the responsibilities towards their children. People who have adopted children are also parents, and foster parents take care of children on behalf of their biological parents.

Why do my parents treat me as if I am still a baby?
The relationship between a parent and a teenage child is often challenging. The reason for this is that the teenage or adolescent years represent the stage between being a child and being an adult. You want more independence, but your parents know the dangers that lie in the big outside world, and probably want to protect you from harm.

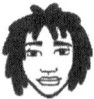

Why are my parents so behind the times?
The world has changed very fast in the last twenty or thirty years: attitudes and behaviour, fashions, education, technology, politics, music, etc. Perhaps you have decided your parents are old-fashioned without even trying to let them explain why they like something or want to do something. Have you tried to talk openly about it to them?

***My parents don't understand how difficult it is to be a teenager.
How can I get them to listen?***

There are no hard and fast rules for parental relations with teenagers.
Every family will have different priorities, and principles and moral values
will differ from one family to another. The important rules for good relationships between parents and teenagers are trust, mutual respect* and
openness. If you feel too shy to talk to your parents, or feel they won't
understand or will be critical, try to find another adult to talk to and discuss your feelings with them.

Remember you are feeling your way into an adult world and your parents are feeling their way into being responsible for a teenager. Don't cut
them out.

Consider discussing your ideas with an aunt or uncle or the parents of
a friend, where there is less emotion at stake, so that when you come to
talk to your own parents you have a clearer head and a better understanding of the issues from an adult's point of view.

Why are my parents so strict?

Because they love you! At least in most cases this is the reason why. In
their own lives they will have experienced the pains of growing up, and
this will often make them over-protective. Parents, in general, don't want
their kids to get hurt. On the other hand, teenagers often feel that they
want to experience the world and learn from their own mistakes, and this
can lead to tension and conflict.

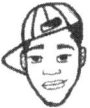

What are my parents' rights over me?

Until you are 18 you are legally a minor and the responsibility of your parents. Furthermore, until you leave home you are dependent on them for
your keep. So certain ground rules have to be worked out, e.g. regarding
clothes, allowances, boyfriends*/girlfriends*, drinking, music, clubbing, homework, late nights, working, etc. You need to agree together on the rules so
that you and your parents can agree to abide by them.

How can I get my parents to allow me more freedom?

Your need for independence is probably in conflict with your parents' need
to enforce limits and discipline. It is important to remember that in order
to be treated as an adult you must first act in an adult manner. The way
to get your parents to give you greater autonomy is to show them that
you can be responsible while being independent.

The world in which our parents grew up was very different from your own, and your parents probably want to protect you from what they see as a dangerous modern world, riddled with violence, sex, sexually transmitted infections* and drugs*. Show your parents that you respect* them and the rules to which you have agreed and they are likely to treat you with greater respect too.

Do parents have the right to beat their children?

The right to discipline children should never be confused with the physical abuse* of children. Many people would argue that parents do *not* have the moral right to hit their children, especially when they are small, vulnerable, dependent, easily frightened and cannot hit back.

In Zimbabwean law parents do have the right to give their children a hiding, as long as they do not beat them so hard that the child is injured, or that the child is beaten constantly for no reason. If this should happen it would be up to the court to decide whether the beating was serious enough for the parent to be charged with a crime. These laws are not in line with the Convention on the Rights of the Child.

The word 'beat' should not be used lightly. It means hitting someone very hard or in a sustained manner and should not be confused with a smack or slap for bad behaviour.

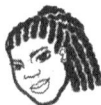

How do I tell my parents that I have a boyfriend*?

Choose a suitable time to talk to your parents, or one of them, when they are relaxed and not busy or tired. Don't mention it in the middle of an argument, or last thing at night. You could start by saying that you are telling them about your boyfriend because you'd rather be honest with them than do something behind their backs. Tell your parents that their acceptance of you having a boyfriend means a lot to you. If you expect an angry reaction you may consider asking an older sibling or family friend to be around when you tell them, or even to tell them on your behalf.

Why can't my boyfriend visit me at home?

Your parents are probably finding it difficult to acknowledge that you are old enough to have a boyfriend. Don't sulk or stop talking to them. Your parents need to be able to trust you and you, in turn, need to earn that trust. Parents need to support and respect teenagers, as well as to give them enough information to make wise decisions.

Try to get your parents to realise that if you do not bring your boyfriend home you might meet in an unsafe place where they might not even know where to find you.

How can I get my parents to trust me?

Trust has to be earned. It does not just happen. Firstly, it is advisable that sexual matters are discussed openly with your parents so that they can advise you. Once you have established clear lines of communication with them, the trust between you should grow. The key to gaining your parent's trust is to be honest with them, instead of being secretive and disobedient. Rather than starting out a relationship with a boyfriend* on a wrong footing, it would be better to adhere to your parents' limits, especially at the beginning. Remember that your parents set limits for your own safety and not to spoil your fun. Usually if parents see that you are being responsible and adhering to their rules, they will trust you more and possibly become more lenient about restrictions. It also helps if your parents know whom you are going out with, so it might be a good idea to introduce your boyfriend to them. Gaining your parents' trust may be a slow and gradual process, but it will be worth it in the end.

How can I get my parents to like my boyfriend?

Nothing that you do will directly influence your parents' like or dislike of your boyfriend. Your parents will form their own opinion, based on their interaction with him. However, talking openly with your parents about the boyfriend will perhaps allow you an opportunity to clarify any wrong impressions that they may have. Similarly, your parents may point out facts about your boyfriend that you did not notice and that you need to think about.

Why are my parents unwilling to talk openly about sex?

Your parents may think that if they speak openly to you about sex you may see it as them giving you permission to be sexually active. They may also be unsure of how you will react. Your parents may fear that you might be embarrassed at the mention of sex or sexuality. Parents may also not want to discuss the topic because they are not sure how much their child already knows about it. Don't forget, your parents were children once and their parents probably did not talk to them either.

Try to take the initiative. Find the right occasion to bring up the subject, try to do it gently and politely, try to explain that you would like advice, or that you would like to know what people thought when *they* were growing up, or what *they* felt when they first went out on a date. Usually parents welcome it when their son or daughter talks to them. They feel trusted rather than excluded from your life and ideas and will want to talk more freely.

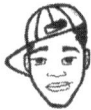

Should I tell my parents who I've slept with?

Usually it isn't a good idea to share details of your sex life with your parents. Just as you probably wouldn't want to hear details of your parents' sex life! Your parents may struggle to accept that you are a sexual human being. Certain parent-child boundaries are important and should be respected.

Do I have to respect my parents or should they earn that respect*?

Your parents gave you life, cared for you and support you. For this reason alone it is your duty and obligation to respect them. On the other hand, your parents should provide a good example to you in order to nurture your respect. Remember your parents are human beings too: they will, therefore, sometimes get tired, upset, worried or irritated; wear the wrong clothes at an important function, ask silly questions of your friends and so on. Try to be tolerant and understanding – no one is perfect!

Why does my father never do household chores?

Traditionally fathers never cooked or did household chores because as children they were told that certain things are done by girls and certain things are done by boys. For example, girls were supposed to help their mothers in the kitchen, clean the house and help look after their siblings. Boys were supposed to help their fathers in the shop, if they were shopkeepers, or look after the cattle, if they were herders, cut the wood, and so on.

Today, in modern society, we see men and women as equal citizens, because the role of women has changed so much. Women now also work outside the home to earn an income. So it has become necessary to revise the traditional roles of men and women. Everybody, male or female, has something to offer and each family will work out its own system of dividing the household chores. The most sensible way is to share the tasks which no one likes doing very much, so that the same person does not end up doing them. It will also give everybody a chance to learn new skills!

If your dad is too set in his ways to change let him be, but make sure that your brother is not spoilt in the same way.

Why does my father make all the decisions in our household?

Fathers traditionally believed that they were the heads of the household, the main breadwinners and therefore had the right to be the final authorities, even sometimes over kitchen matters. More modern families try to ensure that there is equality and respect* between both parents and that all decisions are discussed and agreed upon together.

If you live in a family where the father is the final authority over everything it is probably best not to argue too much, because you can't win. You can, however, support your mother by helping her, and you can decide that when you have your own family you will make sure that there is more respect and equality between you and your partner. Legally mothers and fathers are equal, and neither has a greater right to make decisions.

Why is my mother so subservient to my father?

Many women are submissive because as little girls they were told not to question their father's decisions, and taught to obey their husbands. Their brothers may also have been treated in a way that made them feel superior to their sisters. In addition, many religions* teach that wives should be obedient to their husbands.

However, women have a right to their own opinions, and to say what they feel. One person or one gender* should not be exploited to the advantage of the other. Because it was often different in the past, it is up to the young men and women of today to show each other mutual respect and learn to base their opinions on sound reasons that they can discuss.

Why do some parents molest* their children?

About 30% of parents who molest their children have been molested or sexually abused as children themselves, quite often by a close relative. Usually the molester was not believed when, as a child, he or she tried to tell someone about their own sexual abuse*; or was too frightened to tell another adult, because they knew they would not be believed.

If a parent rapes* a child this is a terrible abuse of trust and may have a devastating effect on that child's life, in the present and the future.

Will I turn out to be like my father?

Not necessarily. You share a genetic pool – in other words, you will certainly inherit some physical and psychological characteristics – but you are a different person who can make choices of your own. If there are things about your father which you admire and respect you will want to follow his example. If there are attitudes and behaviour which you dislike or despise you can make a conscious decision *not* to behave in this way.

If you feel you are behaving in a way that you don't want to, and you think that it is because of inherited characteristics, you may need some counselling and guidance to help you become stronger and change your behaviour.

Rather than sit at home and worry, try to find someone to talk to about your concerns – maybe a sympathetic teacher.

Paternity see Fatherhood

Patriarchal society

A patriarchal society is one in which power is held by older men, and women, who are given different roles, are often treated as junior partners or children. All social practices are arranged for the convenience of the men. Some traditional African societies, as well as some Muslim societies, as well as most traditional European societies, are patriarchal. There are many remnants of patriarchal attitudes in modern societies. Men still dominate in many arenas, particularly politics.

What are the characteristics of a patriarchal society?

Despite the enormous changes in the second half of the previous century as regards the role of women, many people still think that we are living in a man's world: that men have more power and authority, and that women have less say and are not valued as highly as men. Since 1994 various laws have been passed in South Africa to try to bring patriarchy to an end. To discriminate against women in public life and the workplace is now against the law.

However, some families still see the man as the 'head of the household', even if the woman contributes equally to the income and does more of the housework. They therefore still think that if there is only enough money to send one child to school it should be the boy, even though his sister might be cleverer and keener to get an education*. This is wrong. All children should be given the same opportunities.

'Women constitute half the world's population,
perform nearly two-thirds of its work hours,
receive one-tenth of the world's income,
and own less than one-hundredth of the world's property. UN REPORT

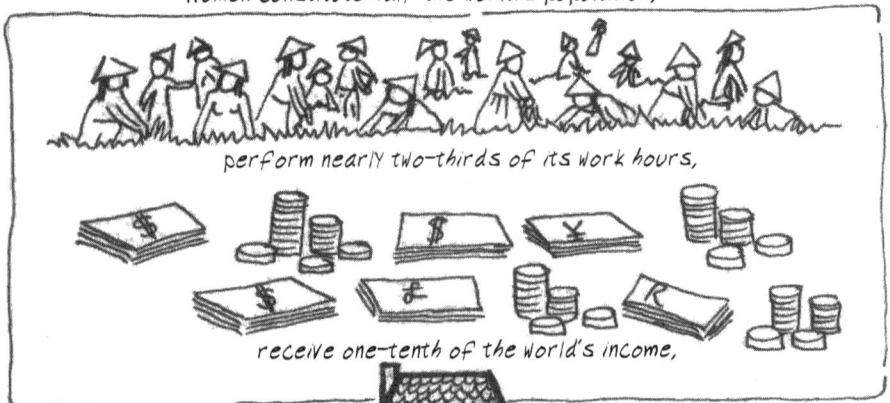

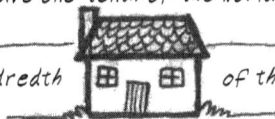

Peer pressure

Peer pressure is the strong influence exerted by persons your own age on you to do things in order to be part of the group. Being a teenager is a time when we experiment with new things. Quite often you may not wish to do these things, but you do so in order to be accepted and not excluded by your group. For example, very often teenagers engage in early sexual relations because of pressure from their group and not because they feel they are ready for it. It is the same with taking drugs* or smoking* or drinking alcohol*, which you feel pressured to do because your peers make you believe that it is cool to do these things.

Why is it so difficult to resist peer pressure?
Peer pressure is difficult to deal with, because you don't want your peers to tease you or despise you because you won't conform; and you may not want to, for example, drink or smoke. But remember, peer pressure is all about conformity. It is all about the security of everyone doing the same thing, even if it is not the right thing to do. In other words, even the people who are leaning on others to join in are not as self-confident as they might seem.

People who learn to resist peer pressure when young tend to do better later in life, because they have learnt not to be pushed around and they know what they want, and do not feel ashamed of their decisions.

How do I resist peer pressure?
Don't follow the example of your peers blindly. Learn to make up your own mind, especially about important matters such as sex, drugs, smoking and alcohol.

You need to *know* yourself before you can *be* yourself and be true to what you believe in. Don't do something you don't feel like doing. Dare to be different from others when you do not agree with them. It takes more courage to be different than to conform. When something doesn't feel right it is never a good idea to go along just because everyone else is doing so.

It's also a good idea to talk about peer pressure with an adult or friend that you trust. Discuss what you would do in different situations where there might be peer pressure. That way you will be better prepared to deal with the real-life situation when it happens. For example, if you discuss your feelings and opinions about sex with someone you trust you will discover what your values are around sex. Then, if you are in a situation where you feel pressured to have sex, you will be able to say 'no' if you don't want to, because you've already decided that you don't believe in having sex until you're older.

Peer pressure is very much part of a teenager's life; it's unavoidable, so try to be clear about what you want to and will do. Set boundaries for yourself – for example, that you will have one beer but not five.

Ironically, if you show independence you are more likely to gain respect[*] than to be excluded from the group you wish to join.

Penis

The male sex organ, informally also called 'cock', 'prick' or 'dick'. The penis is part of the male reproductive system.

Does the size of one's penis determine how good sex will be?
No. This is a myth that is unproven. Sex can be satisfying irrespective of the size of the penis.

Why are men so concerned about the size of their penises?
It's a myth that all men are penis-fixated. However, quite a few are indeed fixated on the penis. They boast about it being big, and if it is small they feel inadequate. Many men assume that women think that men with small penises cannot satisfy a woman sexually. It may be true in some cases, but for very many women sex is not about penis size but about how sensitive their partner is to a woman's needs. And for many men too sensitivity is more important than the size of their organ.

Why do penises differ in size?
Just like other physiological differences, such as tall and short, fat and thin, the physical build of a particular person determines his penis size. Of necessity penis size has to differ from person to person.

Physical abuse see Abuse

Pimp

A pimp is someone who acts as a go-between between sex workers[*] (prostitutes) and customers. The pimp takes a large percentage of the payment.

Polygamy

Also see **Marriage**

Polygamy is a system of marriage whereby a man can have more than one wife or a woman can have more than one husband. Specifically, when a man has more than one wife it is known as polygamy. In southern Africa it is sometimes part of both African and Muslim tradition to practise that form of polygamy where a man has more than one wife. While African polygamous marriages are now recognised by law, Muslim polygamous marriages are not yet recognised.

Pornography

Pornography is the explicit portrayal or description of people taking part in sexual activity, which can be found in magazines, books, films and videos. Pornography is used to arouse sexual excitement and erotic feelings.

In South Africa possession of pornography is not illegal, except in the case of child pornography – which is punishable by law.

Pregnancy

This nine-month period (40 weeks or 280 days) is known as the 'gestation period'. It is the period of time required by a mother to allow her body to develop the baby until it is able to function for itself outside her body. Thus during this time all the baby's major organs are developed and strengthened to enable the baby to survive on its own.

What are the signs of pregnancy?
Generally the tell-tale symptoms are that the woman ceases to menstruate* and has frequent bouts of nausea or morning sickness*. To know for sure, she needs to go for a pregnancy test.

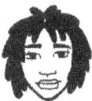

Can a woman have sex when she is pregnant?
It is perfectly normal to have sex when you are pregnant, at least until it becomes too uncomfortable for the woman. Having sex does not hurt or place the baby at risk in any way.

Can my girlfriend* become pregnant if she has sex during her period?
No, she cannot become pregnant while she is menstruating. However, hygienically it is not a good time to engage in sexual activity.

Are there easier ways than using contraception* to prevent pregnancy?

No. There are many myths about ways to prevent yourself from getting pregnant, e.g. eating blotting paper, taking aspirin, drinking coke with aspirin, rinsing your private parts with lemon juice, etc. They are all nonsense. The only way to prevent pregnancy is to take proper precautions.

What happens to unmarried girls who find themselves pregnant? Where can they go for help?

If she is over 18 and loves the father of the baby, they may decide to get married. If she does not want to marry the father and her family supports her, she may decide to have the baby and bring it up with the help of the family. Some girls have the baby but then give it up for adoption*. In South Africa abortion* is legal, so a pregnant girl who feels that she cannot cope with having a baby can go to a family planning clinic, hospital or doctor for advice.

Some girls who do not have these options try to abort, others dump or abandon their babies (baby dumping*) and some commit suicide* or try to do so, because they cannot bear the shame that comes with the pregnancy if they have no family or no partner to support them. Although society has become more tolerant and understanding in many ways, there is still often a stigma attached to an unmarried (and abandoned) mother. As an alternative to suicide a girl may place herself at risk by subjecting herself to a back-street abortion that could result in her death. Finally, she may choose to dump or kill her baby once it has been born.

Such drastic measures should not be considered. Organisations such as Childline* offer advice and help to girls in trouble. Phone them if there is no one else that you can talk to or take into your confidence. Before considering anything drastic, like suicide, speak to someone mature and get advice.

What happens to unmarried girls in traditional societies who fall pregnant?

Customs and traditions vary a good deal. But we can say that tradition in southern Africa requires that when an unmarried girl becomes pregnant she must tell her family, and she may do this by telling her aunt. The male elders will have to come together and take the girl to the boyfriend's home. There they will talk to the elders and discuss the pregnancy and request damages (cattle or other material goods or money). The girl is then cared for by her own family, where the child will be raised.

In African culture, what are the customary steps taken against a man who gets a woman or a girl pregnant when she is not married?
Under customary law, if a man has sexual intercourse* with a girl or woman who is not married and she becomes pregnant the woman's or the girl's family may sue him for damages. This means he will have to make a payment that will compensate for the fact that the family will not be able to charge as high a bride price* when she gets married.

In the case of rape* some families still insist that the perpetrator of the rape must marry the girl he has raped, no matter how young she is, or how old he is, or even whether he already has a wife or not. Traditionally this may have solved the problem, but today rape is seen as a crime of violence. Forcing the girl to marry the man who has raped her may in some societies be seen to restore her honour, but it also often adds to the girl's suffering. This tradition therefore needs to be questioned and challenged.

Rape, forcing a girl to have sex against her will, is not a sign of love* or respect*. Some men still argue that wanting to have sex with a woman or girl, even against her will, shows how attractive they find her. This is clearly nonsense.

Are pregnant girls allowed to go to school?

Most schools do not allow girls to come to school while they are visibly pregnant. They feel that girls who have fallen pregnant set a bad example to others. That means that the education* of girls who fall pregnant while at school gets interrupted or stops altogether.

Historically if a girl fell pregnant she was penalised by not being allowed to continue with her education. Education authorities were, like today, afraid that pregnant learners would send out the wrong message to others. The boy who made her pregnant was not penalised in a similar fashion, although this is now being reviewed in Zimbabwe. There is nothing to prevent a pregnant girl continuing with her education today in South Africa. In Zimbabwe, although constitutionally a pregnant student should be allowed to continue with her education, in practice this rarely happens. Obviously additional care and attention will be required as she will have parental responsibilities to cope with once the baby is born.

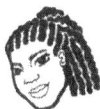

What should I do if I happen to fall pregnant while still at school?

Pregnancy in such a situation is an anxious and often lonely time. The first thing to do is to talk to an adult you trust. If there isn't one you should call Childline* and seek their advice and support.

If you are happy to be pregnant and look forward to having the baby, go to a doctor for a check-up. If he confirms the pregnancy you need to look after your health: don't smoke or drink, exercise and eat healthy foods.

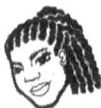

What is diabetes and how does it affect a pregant woman?

Diabetes is a disease in which the sugar and starch (carbohydrates) in your diet* are not properly absorbed into the blood. Diabetics therefore suffer from an imbalance of insulin, a hormone*, which upsets the sugar levels in their bloodstream. It is an illness that has to be controlled carefully by diet and medication. Being diabetic is a risk factor in pregnancy, because if the blood-sugar levels are not controlled it can affect the unborn baby's growth.

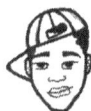

How does high blood pressure during pregnancy affect the mother?

High blood pressure can develop during pregnancy. It usually occurs in first pregnancies and is one of the greatest risk factors for women giving birth. This is why it is very important for a pregnant woman to go for regular ante-natal (before birth) check-ups. That way she will be told early on if she has high blood pressure, and knowing that, she can take care to have it monitored more carefully. High blood pressure is also risky for the unborn baby because it affects the oxygen supply to the foetus.

Can you get pregnant if you have sex only once or have sex standing up?

Most definitely yes, in both cases. You can become pregnant if you have sex only once, or standing up, and do not take precautions. Of course, few people who have sex once expect to become parents!

Who should take responsibility for an unwanted pregnancy?

Usually, both the man and the woman. However, if the man has pressured the woman in any way to have sex with him, or if he has had sex with an under-age girl, then he is responsible. It would be a shared responsibility if the couple engaged in consensual sex, where both agreed.

If the man and the woman chose to have sex and took no precautions and she now finds herself pregnant they both have a responsibility to do the best for the baby they are bringing into this world.

If a single teenage girl finds herself to be pregnant she has to decide whether she is going to go ahead with the pregnancy. This decision can depend on religious, moral, practical and financial circumstances. Because she is not married to the father he has no legal rights over the baby, but he should still pay maintenance, and ideally should be involved in decisions relating to the baby.

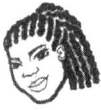

How do parents* react to teenage pregnancies?

It varies from parent to parent. However, most parents want the very best for their children. Most do not want their daughters to become pregnant when they are still teenagers because they know that looking after a baby or children is not easy, and will inevitably interrupt their education*.

Many parents still feel that sex before marriage is wrong, and they are ashamed to think that their own child might be considered by people to have 'loose morals' or that they have not brought him or her up 'the right way'. They will also somehow feel guilty for allowing this to happen. Ultimately, however, most parents, once they have worked through their own feelings, will want to give their daughter and the child support. Often when a teenage girl becomes pregnant it is the mother or grandmother who is left holding the baby – who has to care for it.

Teenage boys are sometimes quite irresponsible. They will deny that they fathered the child and may accuse the mother of 'sleeping around'. If they adopt this attitude it is important to have the support of your own parents, and this will mean being very honest with them.

If you feel very alone, and don't know how to tell your parents, there are advice centres in both Zimbabwe and in South Africa for girls who become pregnant when they are still at school, and they will provide you with advice and counselling.

Pre-menstrual tension (PMT)

Pre-menstrual tension (PMT) is a condition that occurs in some women and girls for several days before menstruation* due to the release of hormones* into their bodies, and the build-up of water and salt. This causes some women to be tense, irritable, weepy – emotions which have a physical cause but may spill over in other situations. Women with PMT need to recognise their condition and not blame themselves for their emotions, and they need sympathy from others. Some women also develop headaches. In extreme cases a doctor may prescribe medication to overcome or reduce PMT.

Progesterone

Progesterone is the female hormone responsible for preparing the inner lining of the womb (the uterus)* for pregnancy.

Proposition

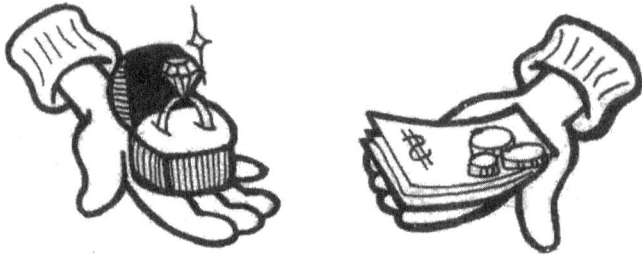

What is the difference between being proposed to and being propositioned?

When the word 'propose' is used in relationships it usually means an offer of marriage* and it is usually accompanied by statements of undying love*. To proposition someone is a way of suggesting a deal: sex for money. A man (or sometimes a woman) will proposition a sex worker* for money, or vice versa. If you are not a sex worker and someone propositions you you can take it as an insult if you like, and behave accordingly; or you can simply treat it with the contempt it deserves.

Prostitution see Sex workers

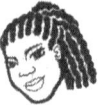

What causes people to become prostitutes?

Prostitutes are people who in return for payment offer their bodies for sexual intercourse*. Most prostitutes are women. In very poor societies this may be the woman's only means of her own or her children's survival. There would, however, be no prostitutes, or sex workers as they are more generally known today, if there were no men who are prepared to pay for sex.

This is another aspect of society where there is often a lot of hypocrisy: women are 'bad', men are 'irresponsible'. Some men will even say, 'I always pay prostitutes as little as I can, because I don't think they should be encouraged.'

Children and young people can be forced into prostitution against their will. They may be brought into a country (trafficking) by syndicates who pretend that they are going to give them proper jobs and who then force them into the sex trade. In such cases they are usually in an unknown country illegally, very often they don't speak the language, and they are threatened by the syndicate. Thus it is a terrible form of slavery.

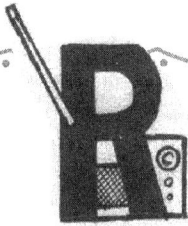

Rape

Rape is committed when a man or boy forces a woman or girl to have sexual inter-course* without her consent. The man's penis* must touch the woman's genitals (the vulva*) but does not have to enter the vagina*. Legally, a woman cannot rape a man; she can only be charged with rape if she holds down a woman to be raped by a man or assists with a rape in some other way. This is called 'assisted rape' and it is a crime for which she can be charged. When a man forces another man to have anal sex*, e.g. in prison, it is another form of rape.

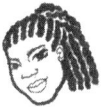

Are women responsible for being raped?
Women have been made to believe that the way they dress or the way they behave are reasons why rape occurs. However, these factors can-not possibly point towards any blame on the part of the woman. Irre-spective of how a woman dresses or behaves (her fundamental human rights), she is very rarely responsible for being raped. If a woman refuses to have sexual intercourse she is within her legal right to do so. Rape can-not be justified by pointing to how a woman was behaving or how she was dressed. Rapists will usually want to blame someone other than them-selves. They will often aggressively insist that it was the victim's fault, because, for example, she was wearing a short skirt. This is a smokescreen to hide the fact that someone has behaved in a violent and immoral way, and has had no control over his emotions.

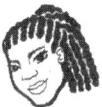

Can your partner rape you?
If you refuse sexual relations with your partner but your partner contin-ues and forces you to engage in sexual intercourse, then it is rape. Many women incorrectly believe that a husband or boyfriend* cannot be charged with rape. If you do not consent to sexual intercourse, irrespective of who the partner is, he can be charged with rape.

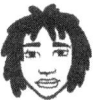

How is rape punished by law?
The rape of a woman or a child is considered a serious criminal offence. A person convicted of rape in a court of law can be sentenced to prison

for not less than five years, and it may be more than twenty years, depending on the circumstances. In Zimbabwe if you are convicted of rape you can be tested for HIV* without your consent. If you are found to be infected with HIV your sentence can be longer.

People who have been raped are often afraid to give evidence in court, especially if they have to look at the person who raped them. As a result, both South Africa and Zimbabwe are introducing special courts where rape victims can give evidence in private, where they may be able to speak more freely. This helps to make sure the rapist is convicted (found guilty). During the last decade the legal systems in these two countries have undergone reform, allowing children too to give evidence in a less intimidating environment.

Since people charged with crimes cannot be punished until the court finds them guilty, rapists are often released on bail until their trial takes place. In order to protect a rape victim she may be taken to a special home where she can be safe from the accused person until after the trial. Some people believe that men or boys accused of rape should not be let out of prison on bail, but the law still allows them to be.

Very often the first thing a raped woman does is to throw away items of clothing that might have been torn or soiled. Remember, should you ever be raped keep all clothes and hand them to the police, as they can be used in evidence against the perpetrator.

Can one get HIV or STIs* from being raped?

Sexually transmitted infections, including HIV, are frequently passed to a woman or a girl during rape. If the victim is a child it often is not discovered until much later, as the child may not understand what has happened and may be afraid to tell anyone. Moreover, a perpetrator, especially if it is a family member, tends to threaten his young victim: do not tell your mother or something dreadful will happen to you.

Having an STI is often the way in which the offence is first discovered.

One consequence of the AIDS* pandemic is that some men believe the only way to have sex 'safely' is to have it with a virgin. This, of course, is nonsense, because they can use a condom*. Instead, the young woman is forced to have sex, and will often suffer irreparable damage.

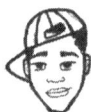

Can males also be raped?

Yes. Males can be victims of sodomy* – anal sex*. It is something that can happen in prisons where younger men are raped by older men. In Zimbabwe any non-consensual sex is regarded as rape and the perpetrator can be punished. Rape of both women and men is now recognised internationally as a weapon of war, and as a consequence people can be tried for rape by an international war crimes tribunal.

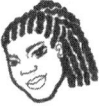

Where can I go for help should I ever be raped?

Depending on the particular circumstances and what is closer you should either go to your nearest hospital or police station. It is imperative that you do not bath before you go, as this will wash off all the evidence. And if you have torn or soiled clothing this should be preserved in a brown paper bag to be used as evidence. (Do not use a plastic bag as it will affect the forensic examination.) At the police station or hospital a statement will be taken and a thorough examination conducted in order to obtain the necessary medical evidence required to identify the accused and to satisfy the necessary legal requirements to take the matter to court.

What can one do to prevent being raped?

Try to remain in a crowd and avoid being completely alone with any man. Even if the man is a good family friend and you've known him since you were little. Be extremely careful and act responsibly at all times.

What exactly is 'statutory rape'?

This is a phrase that confuses many people, because it is not actually rape. It is the term used for the crime that is committed when a person over the age of 16 has sexual intercourse[*] with a girl under the age of 16 after she has consented. It is also called 'under-age sex'. No force is used. It is a crime because the girl will not have reached the age of legally being able to consent to sex. A person who commits statutory rape may be sentenced to prison or may be fined, depending on the circumstances.

Religion

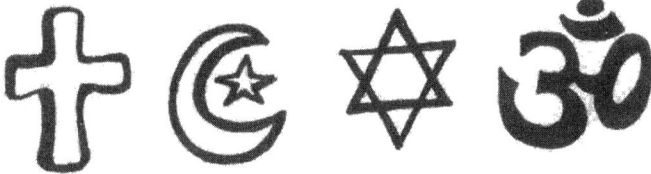

All cultures have some form of religion. Each religion promotes a way of life and a set of values and practises a form of worship of a higher being. Not all members of a culture practice its religion or adhere to the teachings to the same extent.

If someone has no firm conviction for or against a particular religion that person is an agnostic. Someone who firmly believes there is no higher being is called an atheist.

Is religion the same thing as culture?

Often culture and religion go together, but not necessarily. In the same country and culture you can find people belonging to different religions. In India, for example, you find Hindu, Muslim as well as Christian Indians. In the same way you can find Jews who are atheist or Christian.

Should religion affect my relationship with a boyfriend*?

Religion can play a very big part in how you conduct your relationship. Any religion will lay down the moral ground rules for behaviour with the opposite sex. The depth of your belief will determine the extent to which religion will influence your relationship.

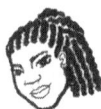

If my partner is not Christian, do I have the right to insist that my child be brought up as one?

Of course you have a right to want a religious upbringing for your child. Religion is an important anchor in the life of a child as it provides the child with early moral principles that will remain throughout his or her life. The decision as to which religion the child will follow must be taken after rational discussion by both parents* who have a joint responsibility in making this decision. You cannot impose your religion on your child without consulting with your partner.

Remember that this is one of many important issues that you should be aware of during courtship, which is a period of discussion and exploration. If there are huge differences of opinion about certain issues, and they are not resolved, these may affect the happiness of your marriage* and of your children.

What role should African beliefs play in my life?

Custom and beliefs are an essential part of our upbringing. However they should not be followed blindly or thoughtlessly. It is necessary for you to discuss and assess the various beliefs in order to ascertain whether they infringe on any of your basic human rights. If they do, then these are beliefs that should not be adopted into your life. Remember that as human beings we can choose what values and principles to adopt, and we must learn to take responsibility for our decisions.

Reproductive organs

The **male reproductive system** consists of those organs that enable the man to fulfil his reproductive function – in other words, to produce sperm*, have sexual intercourse*, ejaculate*, and supply sperm that can fertilise an ovum in the Fallopian tube of the woman.

Sperm is produced in the testes• due to the influence of hormones*, stored in the seminal vesicle• and released into the woman's vagina* during sexual intercourse. From there the spermatozoons• move to the woman's uterus and into the Fallopian tubes, where they might encounter an ovum• and one may penetrate and fertilise it.

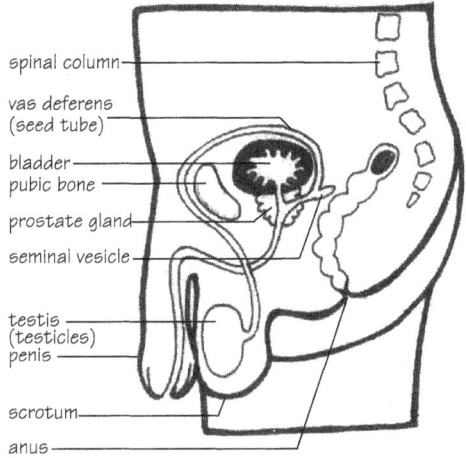

spinal column

vas deferens (seed tube)

bladder
pubic bone

prostate gland

seminal vesicle

testis (testicles)
penis

scrotum

anus

The **female reproductive system** consists of those organs that make it possible for the woman to fulfil her reproductive function – in other words, to ovulate, have sexual intercourse, contain and feed a fertilised ovum (egg)• inside her body until the foetus is ready to be born, and then to give birth* to a baby. Except for the vulva (the exterior sex organs), the woman's reproductive organs are all situated in the pelvis (the basin-shaped cavity between the hip bones).

Usually only one ovum is released each month during ovulation*. The ovum is released by one of the two ovaries• into a Fallopian tube•. If the ovum meets up with a sperm on its way to the uterus• and the sperm penetrates the ovum fertilisation happens. The fertilised ovum immediately starts dividing and changes into a little ball consisting of many small cells. When this little ball reaches the uterus, it becomes implanted in the lining and changes into an embryo•, then a foetus, and finally a baby. Also see the diagram on page 101.

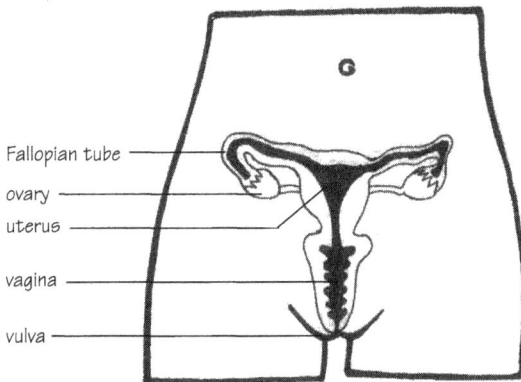

Fallopian tube

ovary

uterus

vagina

vulva

R

Respect

An attitude of admiration; to show consideration and treat courteously.

Do I have a duty to respect my elders?

Elders have lived longer than we have and have therefore learnt a lot more than we have. In the light of this it is important that we give them the respect they deserve, based on their greater age and experience. However, if someone's behaviour is consistently immoral, careless, hurtful or violent, no one has a duty to respect them simply because they are older.

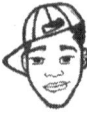

How do I show respect to my parents*?

As you grow up respect between parent and child is essential for a healthy relationship. It is important that you listen and assess your parents' views on all sorts of issues: education, politics, relationships, religion, your future career – even sport and music! Remember that your parents have greater experience and that you may be able to learn from them. The greatest respect we can give to our parents is to treat them well, be helpful and polite around the house and to allow them to assist us in the growing-up process by taking their well-meant advice seriously.

My father is an alcoholic and he beats my mother. Must I still respect him?

Respect is born of trust, understanding, honesty and wisdom. If your father is consistently drunk and abusive you are more likely to fear rather than respect him, and he will probably remain a bad memory all your life. If there is an older family member whom you love and respect you should discuss the problem with him or her, and if not you should phone Childline* and discuss the issue with a counsellor.

So

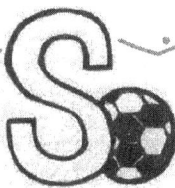

Safe sex see **Contraception**

Sex workers

'Sex workers' is the more current or respectful term for 'prostitutes'. This profession is considered 'the oldest in the world', which indicates that there has always been a demand for women providing sex in exchange for money. Some women choose to become sex workers, or more correctly, some women work in the sex trade, choose to earn money when few other career options may be open to them. Some women are forced into prostitution* by poverty; only by 'selling' their bodies can they and their children survive.

In some countries (e.g. the Netherlands) sex work is taxable and non-criminal and brothels are registered.

Sexual harassment

Also see **Abuse, Molesting**

Sexual harassment is any unwanted behaviour that infringes on the privacy of, or humiliates, a person on the basis of sex, or is intended to persuade someone to submit to sexual advances. It often happens in the workplace or educational institutions. It may come from a person in a position of greater power or authority, but not necessarily. There are many different forms of sexual harassment. It can take the form of a male or female boss putting pressure on a subordinate to date or to engage in sex with the underlying threat of losing a job or not getting a promotion if the employee should refuse. Or it could be insulting words or looks or brushing against someone in a sexually suggestive way.

In South Africa sexual harassment is prohibited by law. In Zimbabwe it is dealt with under the new labour law and is defined as an 'unfair labour practice'!

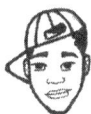

What does groping mean?
To fondle or attempt to fondle a woman's breasts or buttocks, or a guy's genitalia. This is usually a form of harassment and you could be charged if found guilty. Groping is different from fondling which is pleasurable and agreed upon by both people involved. Both can involve the same body parts.

Sexual intercourse

The act of having sex, when a man's penis* enters the body of his partner, usually resulting in ejaculation* and orgasm*, with or without the intention of procreation (to create a baby). Sexual intercourse usually occurs between two consenting adults who in this way express their sexual desire for each other.

Is sexual intercourse defined only in terms of penetration?
Strictly speaking, yes – although foreplay*, heavy petting* and oral sex* are all part of sexual activity.

Whom do I approach if I experience pain when I have sexual intercourse?
See a doctor or a health worker.

Sexually transmitted infections (STIs)

STIs are Sexually Transmitted Infections, i.e. infections transmitted by intercourse. STIs include HIV/AIDS*, genital herpes (small blisters around the mouth or genitalia), syphilis (ulcers and lesions) and gonorrhoea (infection, pain, pus). STIs will eventually damage the nervous system and may cause sterility, or may affect the unborn baby if a woman is pregnant. An STI must be treated by a medical practitioner as soon as it is detected.

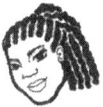

Are there cures for STIs?
If caught early enough, and if the patient is not infected with HIV/AIDS*, penicillin and various antibiotics can cure STIs. If you think you have an STI go to a clinic or doctor as quickly as possible. The best precaution against STIs is not to have unprotected sex.

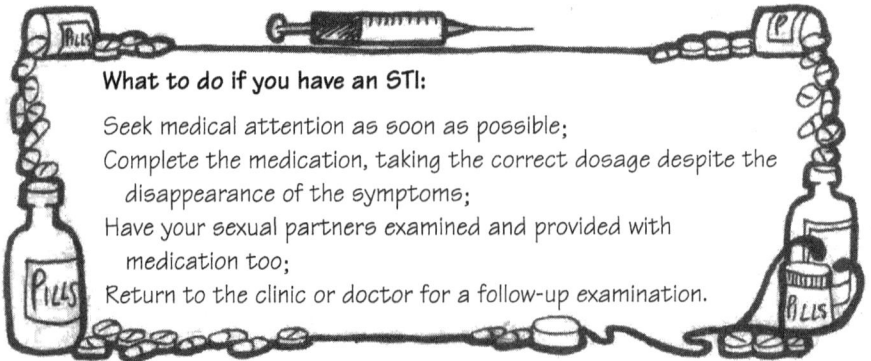

What to do if you have an STI:

Seek medical attention as soon as possible;
Complete the medication, taking the correct dosage despite the disappearance of the symptoms;
Have your sexual partners examined and provided with medication too;
Return to the clinic or doctor for a follow-up examination.

Single mothers

Single mothers are women without partners who, for a variety of reasons, have babies and raise them on their own. The most common reason is that the father of the child refuses to marry or live with or support the woman. In other cases, single mothers are widowed or divorced* women. Increasingly, however, women are choosing to be single mothers because they feel that the men they know are so irresponsible that they are better off without them.

Is it easy to raise a baby on your own?

Women who have babies, but who are not married to the man who is, or acts, as the children's father, often experience great difficulty in raising their children. Making money, supporting themselves and a child or children all alone is hard. The fact that many people still discriminate against such women because they feel that these women do not have the necessary support systems for rearing the children makes it even harder. Some employers feel that single mothers may be unreliable workers as they may have to be absent from work when a child falls ill.

On the other hand, mature single women who prefer their independence and have good jobs that enable them to support a child and provide the necessary child care may decide that they are better off on their own. In such circumstances children are rarely disadvantaged and often have the benefit of a close, stable relationship with their mother. They do, however, lack a male role model, and may suffer from that all their lives.

Smoking

'Smoking' usually refers to the smoking of tobacco, so 'No Smoking' means the smoking of cigarettes* and cigars is prohibited. Smoking of tobacco is addictive* and harmful to one's health.

Other substances too are smoked: *dagga*, marijuana, *mbanje* – all names given to the *Cannabis* plant, which grows naturally in many parts of southern Africa and which has a hallucinogenic effect on the smoker. In Zimbabwe it is illegal to smoke *mbanje* and people can be sentenced to up to ten years in prison for dealing in it. Smoking and dealing in *dagga* is also illegal in South Africa.

Why do people smoke?

Persons smoke for a variety of reasons, e.g. to relieve stress or to lose weight. Many young people smoke because of peer pressure* and wanting to be part of the crowd.

Why is smoking unhealthy?

Smoking is strongly linked to many common cancers – cancer of the lungs, the bladder, the breasts, the cervix and other organs. Research has also proven that the long-term effects of smoking cigarettes* can lead to emphysema and the premature ageing of the skin. In addition people who smoke experience more back and neck pain and recover more slowly from injuries.

Cigarettes contain nicotine, which is inhaled and absorbed into the body through the lungs. As nicotine is addictive, the body becomes dependent on it.

Why are there rules and regulations about smoking in public?

When you smoke you are also affecting other people around you. If somebody smokes in your company you too inhale the fumes. This is called 'passive smoking', and it is unhealthy for the same reasons as normal smoking. In fact, some researchers say passive smoking is more harmful to your health than 'active' smoking.

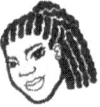

Does smoking harm an unborn baby?

Yes, very much so. Research has shown that babies born to smoking pregnant mothers are adversely affected and can at birth weigh up to half a kilogram less than babies of non-smoking mothers. The toxic substances in cigarettes reach unborn babies through their mothers' blood and they are more susceptible to illness than other babies.

Does smoking reduce sperm* production?

The lungs have no direct connection with the part of your body that produces sperm. Smoking directly affects your lungs and breathing and therefore does not affect your sperm production in any way.

Sodomy

Sodomy is another word for anal sex* with a man or woman. It may be homosexual*, heterosexual or between a man and an animal (bestiality). Sodomy may be consensual, but it has been considered a crime for years in South Africa and in other parts of the world. In Zimbabwe that is still the case if it takes place between two men, even if the men have agreed. It is not a crime if it takes place between a man and a woman and the woman has consented.

If a man forcibly sodomises another man or a woman it is punishable as rape*.

Sperm

Core of ovum

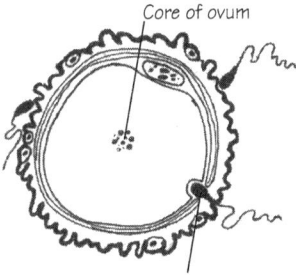

spermatozoon penetrating ovum

Sperm is the male seed that is carried in the semen. Each ejaculation* of semen contains thousands of spermatozoons. Each spermatozoon consists of a big head and a long tail which drives it forward and has a chance of fertilising an ovum or egg in a woman's body. In this way an embryo is created, which develops into a foetus and eventually a baby. Also see the diagram on page 101.

Is my sperm hot when it moves into my girlfriend's vagina*?
No. Your semen, which contains the sperm, is the same temperature as your body and any other body fluid and does not feel hot.

Sterilisation

It is an operation that causes you to become infertile. If a couple has decided that they do not want to have any more children then an operation of this type ensures that the women will not fall pregnant again. After a woman has had 'her tubes tied', as this operation is popularly known, it is unnecessary for her to practise any other form of birth control* – but both Fallopian tubes• must have been tied.

Can men also be sterilised?
Yes, it is called a vasectomy, and in this case the *vas deferens* (seed tubes•) are tied.

Suicide

Suicide happens when a person chooses to end his or her or own life. There are a variety of reasons why people give up on life. They might have been experiencing a deep sense of despair, failure, hopelessness, loss of control, guilt, grief*, even poor health or financial problems. Often people who commit suicide suffer from depression*.

Are there signs that indicate that someone might commit suicide?
Sometimes yes. A very depressed person may be considering suicide – someone who has become withdrawn or who behaves quite unlike his or her usual self. On the other hand, a suicide can be triggered by something as simple as a disagreement, or by the loss of a lover.

How can I stop suicidal thoughts?

Firstly ask yourself: Why am I feeling this way?

Sit still and think why you feel your life is worthless. Do you feel inadequate because you tend to compare yourself to other people? Are these feelings of inadequacy real, or are they only imagined? Why do you feel like a failure? If someone told you this, think carefully whether this is reasonable criticism. Can you truly say about yourself that you have no value as a human being?

The best thing you can do is to talk to someone close to you and try to analyse your feelings and your experiences. Discussing these feelings with a friend may help you to work through these questions and to see yourself in a different light. Counselling by a professional can also help you overcome depression*.

If something has made you so sad that you feel your life has lost its meaning, consider carefully whether the misery is not something which will disappear as time passes. Putting things into words could give you a new perspective, and may help you to see things in a new light and perhaps overcome your sense of grief*.

My sister committed suicide. Why am I feeling guilty about it?

The natural reaction to her suicide is to think that you may have been able to stop her from doing it. You may even fear that some word or action of yours triggered her to take her own life. However, by the time someone decides to commit suicide many things – often minor or unnoticeable to an outsider – would have happened which would have hurt her over a long period. Committing suicide would have been the final act of desperation. For some reason your sister thought the world would be a better place without her, or perhaps she could simply no longer cope with her own feelings. No one will ever really know.

Allow yourself to feel grief, to feel sorrow, to mourn*, to cry. Try to think what you can learn from this experience, because having been through it you have more to offer the world in terms of your own understanding of pain and responsibility.

Think what your sister might have wanted you to do. Surely she would not have wanted to pass her depression on, or wanted you to live with a sense of guilt for the rest of your life. Take life gently, be kind to yourself, write, draw, do anything creative that will help transform the pain from something negative to something positive that you can share with others.

Surrogate mother

A surrogate mother is a woman who agrees to carry the foetus of an unborn baby for another woman. The egg may belong to the surrogate mother or it may belong to the 'donor' mother'. The surrogate mother is acting like an incubator for a baby and the idea is that she gives up the baby at birth to the couple who have contracted her to have it on their behalf. Such arrangements sometimes work out and sometimes don't, as the surrogate mother may change her mind about giving up the baby once it is born. Also the parents* may not fulfil their side of the bargain, and for example refuse to pay her the agreed amount.

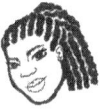

Are there surrogate fathers too?
Yes, if a man agrees to provide sperm* so that another couple can have a child, he is a surrogate father of sorts. This term is however not commonly used for this kind of arrangement. It is rather used to describe a man who acts towards a child like a father, even though there is no biological or legal relationship.

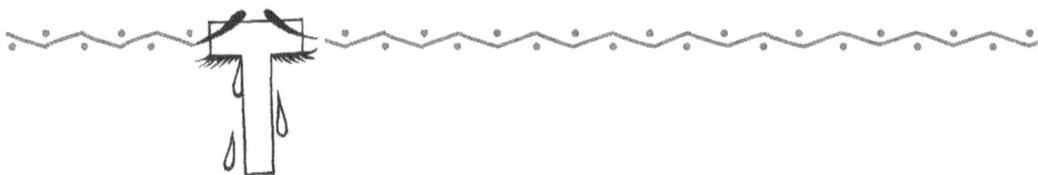

Table manners see Manners

Taboo

A taboo is a cultural or religious value that involves disapproving of a particular practice usually in public, e.g. picking your nose. All cultures have taboos, but these change with time. In Zimbabwe it used to be taboo for a man to hold a woman's hand in public – although holding another man's hand in public was deemed acceptable. In Europe it used to be taboo for a woman to breast-feed in public; today it is generally acceptable.

Taboos are not universal rules against a particular practise. Even within one community or family taboos will differ, especially between the generations. Taboos are useful for regulating society so that people can co-exist peacefully and without causing offence to others, and they help protect people, e.g. from violence or disease. For example, it is taboo for men to urinate against a tree in public in towns, whereas in rural areas it is generally perfectly acceptable.

Taboos only cause problems when they have lost their usefulness and are still rigidly enforced for dubious reasons, usually under the excuse of preserving culture or maintaining standards. For example, at one stage it was taboo to discuss sexual matters with one's parents; in the age of HIV/AIDS* it has become essential.

Teenage pregnancy see Pregnancy

Termination of pregnancy see Abortion

Testosterone

This is the male hormone* that provides men with their male characteristics, even as a foetus and baby, and increasingly during puberty and adolescence. When a young boy becomes a teenager testosterone is released into his body, making him develop into a man: that is why an adolescent boy grows hair on his face and around his genitals, and why his voice grows deeper.

'The Pill' see Contraception

Transsexual, Transgender and Transvestite

These three terms are often confused. A **transsexual** is a person who feels he or she has been born in the wrong body. Many transsexuals undergo sex-reassignment surgery, generally known as a 'sex change'. These operations are possible in South Africa and the person is legally entitled to change their identity documents to reflect their new gender. Sex changes are not possible in Zimbabwe.

A **transgendered person** believes that he or she is psychologically the opposite sex. Unlike transsexuals, transgendered people do not feel that it is necessary to undergo a sex change. Transgendered people often refer to themselves as 'queens'.

Most **transvestites** are heterosexual men. They generally think of themselves as men and perform sexually as men but they are sexually aroused through wearing women's clothing. This can be explained as a form of sexual fetishism (like the wearing of leather or shoes during sex) and psychologists have suggested early conditioning; for example, a man who likes to dress up in a nurse's uniform does so because as a child a certain nurse looked after him nicely.

Trousers

Traditionally it was taboo* for girls and women to wear trousers, because it was seen as disrespectful, and girls wearing trousers were seen as being 'forward' and 'cheeky'. In some churches trousers were regarded as 'men's clothing' and not meant to be worn by women. Some people genuinely believed this; for others the restriction on what women could wear was a form of control, a way of putting 'modern women' down. In some churches today it is still prohibited for women to wear trousers, but to most churches nowadays you can wear whatever you want. Trousers are often prohibited when undergoing certain traditional rituals though.

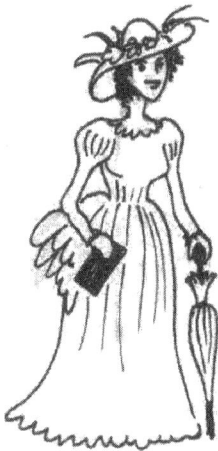

However, when women are performing many of the same physical activities and doing the same jobs as men, trousers or jeans are simply more sensible and practical, just as they are more discreet if, for example, you are climbing a ladder or riding a bicycle.

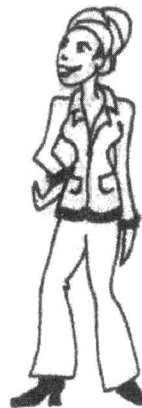

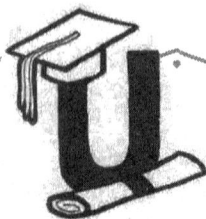

Under-age sex

Sexual intercourse* with anybody under the age of 16 is illegal in Zimbabwe and South Africa, even if the person consents. It is called 'underage sex', and if the partner is over 16 it is considered 'statutory rape' and punishable by law.

Do strong feelings for someone justify under-age sex?
No. Under-age sex is illegal and you can be charged.

Can under-age sex harm a girl physically?
It depends what age you're talking about! Presumably if you're old enough to think about it your body is also sufficiently developed to allow it. But there may be problems of inadequate lubrication (when the vagina is not moist enough) in very young girls, leading to pain and tearing. Although many young girls may appear to be physically ready to engage in sex, they may find it difficult to handle the emotional side of such a sexual relationship. When one is young it is also not wise to get too involved in a relationship as this can prevent you from enjoying your carefree teenage years. So it is better to delay having sex until you are ready for a more permanent relationship and commitment*. What's the rush?

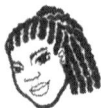

Why can't I have sex before the age of 18?
You can! But why do you want to? You've got the rest of your life after all. It's considered that people under the age of 16 are not mature enough to make rational, informed decisions about what is best for them. The age limit is intended to protect immature young people from being exploited by older, wilier people who may want to take advantage of their innocence. And these days it's better to delay sex, because the longer you wait the less you are at risk of HIV*.

Why can't teachers control their urges with regard to their female students?
It's not that they can't – a few don't want to and the social strictures on this kind of immoral and exploitative behaviour are not powerful enough to put

them off. Until recently teachers in Zimbabwe were not even fired for such an abuse of trust and position, but were simply transferred to another school. This is wrong. Teachers who abuse their authority should be fired and never allowed to work in a school again. The teachers' code of conduct states that in a case of sexual abuse[*] there are grounds for immediate suspension of the teacher, and if he or she is found guilty there are grounds for immediate dismissal. In Zimbabwe a teacher may only be suspended for two years, and may then reapply for his/her position.

If you are harassed by a teacher, tell an adult whom you trust and who will believe what you say. Don't ever think that good grades paid for with your body, and not your brains, are worth it. And if a teacher tells you he loves you and thinks you are beautiful or whatever, *don't* believe him.

Unmarried mothers see **Single mothers**

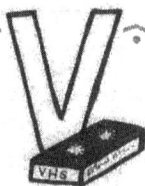

Vagina

The vagina, informally also called the 'fanny' or 'cunt', is part of the female reproductive organs*. It is into the vagina that a male's penis* is inserted in order to engage in sexual intercourse*.

Will my vaginal opening stretch when I have intercourse?
Your vaginal opening will stretch when you have intercourse and return to its normal size afterwards.

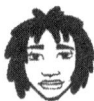

Is it dangerous to put one's finger up a female's vagina?
No. Unless it is a very dirty finger, in which case it will probably be carrying germs.

Is it true that a 'big vagina' spoils sex for men?
No. Size does not matter. In some parts of southern Africa women use herbs to make the vagina dry and tighter – and thus more pleasing to men. This, however, can cause infections and discomfort to the women.

Viagra

Viagra is a medicinal drug designed to help men who have weak or no erections and thus cannot engage in sexual intercourse. It can only be used on prescription from a medical doctor. As is the case with most drugs, it may have side effects and it is necessary to use it as directed.

Virginity

A virgin is someone who has not had full sexual intercourse, although in some societies a girl is only considered to be a virgin if her hymen (a thin membrane covering the opening to the vagina) is unbroken. However, these days, when many girls use tampons and participate widely in sport, the hymen is often not intact when a girl first has intercourse. Sometimes virginity is seen as something to get rid of, but in these days of HIV/AIDS* it is definitely something to hold on to.

Today many people believe that the concept of virginity is sexist, and that virginity testing (practised by some religious sects) is an invasion of the young woman's integrity and her body. Why should women be subjected to this humiliating inspection when men are free to have sex without detection, they ask. They argue that a woman's decision to use her body sexually is her right, and her sexuality should not be controlled by others. Why also is the value of a woman decreased when she loses her virginity whereas the value of a man increases when he loses his. This is a double standard of the worst kind.

My cousin told me that in her church girls are tested for virginity. Is this true?
Yes, sometimes. A certain sect allows that girls as young as three can, and sometimes should, be tested for virginity. The religious elders in the church are supposed to deal with the culprit and resolve the matter, which must never be reported to the police. Usually the girl is made to marry the man who had sex with her as soon as she is old enough to be married.

Such practices are against the law in Zimbabwe and would be considered child abuse[*].

What does 'losing your virginity' mean?
Only a woman who has never engaged in sexual relations with a man can 'lose her virginity'. A woman loses her state of virginity when her hymen, a thin membrane on the inside of the vagina, is ruptured, usually by the insertion of a penis[*]. The expression 'losing your virginity' is thus used to describe what happens when a woman is sexually penetrated for the first time. However, in many women the hymen is torn through other physical activity.

Some people are ashamed to lose their virginity whilst others are proud of it. It all depends on your values and where you are coming from.

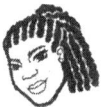

When should I lose my virginity?
Virginity is lost as a normal consequence of engaging in sexual relations. You do not *have* to lose your virginity. You can choose to lose your virginity when you are ready to do so. There is not a right or wrong age for one to lose one's virginity. The choice should be made when you feel you have met a special partner, when you respect each other and are committed to each other. It should be a choice that you feel you want to make. The circumstances should also be right and things like religion[*], morals, family values and cultural background should be considered. If the choice is made to have a sexual relationship, the partners involved must be respon-

sible with regard to protection against pregnancy* and sexually transmitted diseases*, as well as HIV*.

When is the appropriate time to have sex for the first time?

Much of it has to do with emotional preparedness. Don't be pressured by
a partner to do something you don't feel ready for, and make sure there
is some element of commitment* between you. Make sure you're prepared
to avoid pregnancy* and STIs*. Consider having HIV tests if you're not
planning to use condoms*. And if you want to stay a virgin until you get
married – do! Whether you're male or female.

How do I hang on to my virginity?

You need to decide why it is important for you not to have sex. Sometimes
religious values can help you make your decision, but there are other reasons: Why have sex before you are emotionally prepared to do so? Why
not wait until you feel very sure of the guy? Why rush into something that
you can have for decades to come?

 The choice not to have sex is often difficult for teenagers as they have
strong sexual urges and there is generally a fair amount of peer pressure*
to do so. Clear values will help you to not be tempted.

 One way to remain a virgin is to make the decision not to have sex and
then stick with that decision. The issue of sex can be discussed with your
partner, and if he understands your reasons and cares for you he will
support you. If he doesn't, then maybe you are better off without him.

How will people view me if I'm not a virgin? Am I less of a person?

The most important thing is how you will view yourself. Positive self-
esteem does not come with losing your virginity. In fact if the sexual experience was of a bad kind it may even cause you to think less of yourself.
You should not succumb to peer pressure, because eventually you will be
admired for sticking to your own values and morals.

 Films and romantic novels suggest that sex is something wonderful, and
it *can* be between two people who care for each other. But it can also be
a tremendous let-down: 'all that heaving and heavy breathing' can sometimes be a bit painful for a woman the first time round, as well as a bit
frightening. Whether or not you are a virgin is not a criterion by which
you should be judged, or anyone should judge you.

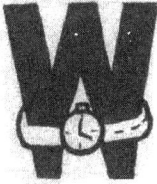

Wedding

There are different types of weddings:

Religious weddings are usually conducted in a church by a priest. This wedding is to comply with the religious requirements of being married.

Formal or **legal weddings** are usually conducted in a formal legal office, such as a registry office or the magistrate's court. The function of this wedding is to comply with the legal requirements of being married.

Traditional or **customary-law weddings** are conducted in the home of the woman. This wedding is to enable parties to comply with the customary-law aspects of marriage*, such as lobola*; or of the formal handing over of the bride from one family to another; or/and of accepting the husband into his wife's family.

Sometimes a couple can get married as many as three times: they might have a quiet registry office wedding, a customary wedding or lobola ceremony and sometimes much later a 'white', or church, wedding.

What is the significance of a wedding cake?

This often highly decorated cake at some weddings represents the high point of the feast, and it is usually cut by the bride and the groom jointly, holding the knife together as a symbol of their first act of married life. Such is the value placed on this act that some couples first have the cake blessed in church.

The cake is often made of dried fruit, because it is something special and lasts. It is often layered in one or two or even more tiers. This is because in some European traditions the second layer of the cake is kept for the first baby's christening.

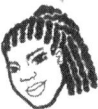

What is the symbolism attached to a wedding ring?

In many traditions the exchange of rings between the bride and the groom symbolises their union and the vows they have made to each other. And the ring, which has no beginning and no end, symbolises unending love.

How are weddings celebrated in other countries?

In most cultures of the world a wedding is a joyful occasion that unites two people and often two families. Every culture will have symbols associated with the wedding. In China, for example, the bride traditionally wears red; in India the occasion lasts three days and includes special ceremonies for both the bride and the groom. In much of Christian Europe the bride wears white (a symbol of purity).

But whatever is worn by the bride, it is often a great occasion for a celebration, a party and for wearing your best clothes.

What is a traditional African wedding ceremony like?

This is a difficult question to answer because traditions vary. However, in a traditional African wedding the ceremony is arranged by the families of both the bride and the groom, after lobola* has been paid to the bride's family. The lobola ceremony can be performed at the homes of both families or only at that of the bride's family. Mostly the bride uses the lobola money to prepare for the wedding.

A traditional wedding takes place at the home of the bride, maybe after a registry-office wedding. The groom's family comes to the bride's home a day before the wedding to be entertained and be welcomed. On the day of the wedding, the bride and groom wear traditional clothes and also perform traditional rituals in the company of people of the same clan and the community at large. The bride is given a new name and she is supposed to bring some new things, such as a bed, dishes, cutlery, and everything else she will need to prepare a meal for her new family the following morning.

If there is a religious wedding as well, the bride, dressed in white, and the groom, in a black suit, will make their vows in the church in the presence of their families and the community. They need a witness to sign the registry, and usually they have matrons of honour, bridesmaids, flower girls, a best man and a pageboy to join them in front of the pulpit. Such a wedding is usually divided into two sessions: first the church ceremony, followed by a reception in a restaurant, church hall or hotel where they might change their outfits.

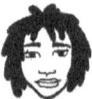

Do we still use waiting rings?

We no longer have waiting rings, although in the past people used beads as a symbol that a particular girl was in a relationship or was going to get married. The beads indicated that no other man could propose to her. The different colours each had a particular meaning, which the community knew.

Wet dreams

Wet dreams are a natural part of a boy's growing-up process. When boys become aware of sexual arousal they dream of sexual intercourse*, resulting in ejaculation* while they are sleeping, as if they were actually having the experience.

Witchcraft

The belief that magical or supernatural powers can be used to cure or to harm people.

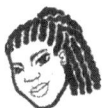

My friend was very upset because when she broke up with her boy-friend* he kept her petticoat and said he would use it to bewitch her. Can this happen?

It is true that undergarments are used by people who believe in the power of witchcraft to put spells on others. Your friend's boyfriend wanted to punish her, but because she had left him he no longer had any say over her. Thus, by keeping her petticoat, he tried to suggest that he still had this power, whereas in reality he did not.

If you really believe something bad is going to happen to you then it generally does, because you will attribute everything that goes wrong to this spell. If you don't believe that you've been bewitched, nothing can hurt you. Good things and bad things happen to most people no matter what they believe.

Support groups and organisations

There are very many organisations and support groups throughout Zimbabwe and South Africa offering services to young people. It is not possible to include them all. We have identified some of the main *drop-in* centres. They in turn will refer you to others when necessary, and give you addresses of their local and regional offices.

ZIMBABWE:

AIDS/HIV support
* **Women and Aids Support Network** provides advice to women living with HIV and AIDS: 13 Walter Hill Avenue, Eastlea, Harare. (04) 791401/2/4
* **The Centre** provides advice and support to people living with HIV: 24 Van Praagh Avenue, Milton Park, Harare. (04) 732965/704728

Abuse
* **Musasa Project** provides support to women and adolescents who have been beaten by their husbands/partners/boyfriends: 64 Selous Avenue, Crn 7th Street, Harare. (04) 794483/725881/4

Alcohol and drug abuse
* **Alcoholics Anonymous** provides support to people who have a drinking problem: 2 Drummond Chaplin Street, Belvedere, Harare. (04) 741770

Child abuse, neglected children and orphans
* **Childline** provides support and advice to children with any kind of problem. Free phone country wide: 961 or Harare (04) 701111/2. They also have a free post service: 60 Livingstone Avenue, Harare.
* **Streets Ahead** provides support to street children: Deseret Centre, Parirenyatwa Hospital, Mazowe Street, Harare. (04) 705074
* **Child Protection Society**. You can write to them for advice; and they try to support children and their families within the framework of children's rights: Box BE 220, Belvedere, Harare. (04) 664370
* **Family Support Trust** provides medical and psycho-social support to victim of abuse and their families: Box SET 506, Southerton, Harare. (04) 668056/7
* **Farm Orphan Support Trust** provides support to the orphans of farmworkers' children: Box Wgt 390, Westgate, Harare. (04) 309800

General support and counselling
* **Samaritans** provides support to people who are feeling lonely and suicidal: 60 Livingstone Avenue, Harare. (04) 722000
* **Connect** gives psychological support and counselling to people and families in need: Box 6298, Harare. (04) 705079
* **Family Support Trust** – see above

Legal advice
* **Legal Aid Directorate** runs a legal advice centre in the Ministry of Justice within the new government complex, Cnr 4th and Samora Machel, Harare. At the time of publication they did not yet have telephones.
* **Zimbabwe Women Lawyers' Association,** 17 Fife Avenue, Harare. Write to them for free legal advice to women and children.

Pregnancy
* **Pregnancy Crisis Centre** provides advice and support to girls and women who have fallen pregnant: No. 6, J. Tongogara Avenue, Harare. (04) 706531

SOUTH AFRICA:

> **Life Line** offers 24-hour emergency counselling on any issue. Consult your local telephone directory for the number closest to you.

Abuse of children
- **Safe Line** is a helpline offering support to abused children: Tollfree 0800 035 553
- **Childline** is a 24-helpline for victims of child abuse: Tollfree 0800 055 555
- The **Child Protection Unit** investigates child abuse and exploitation. Contact your local police for information

AIDS
- **ATICC (Aids Training Information and Counselling Centres)** operate in all major cities: Tollfree 0800 0123 22
- Any local municipal clinic
- **AIDS Helpline** offers advice and counselling to people living with HIV/AIDS: Tollfree 0800 012 322.
- **Love Life** encourages AIDS awareness and promotes healthy living and positive sexuality: Tollfree 0800 121 900

Alcohol and drug abuse
- **Alcoholics Anonymous** offers counselling to abusers of alcohol. Consult your local telephone directory for the number closest to you
- **Tough Love** offers support to families who are victims of drug and alcohol abusers: Cape Town 021 685 5424

Depression and anxiety
- The **Depression and Anxiety Support Group** offers advice to people who suffer from anxiety and depression: Johannesburg 011 7831474
- **Mental Health Society** offers advice to people who suffer from anxiety and depression: Cape Town 021 4479040

Domestic violence
- **Nicro** offers support to both offenders and victims of domestic violence. Consult your local telephone directory for the number closest to you.
- **Live Line** offers support to victims of domestic abuse and referral to relevant organisations: Tollfree 0800 150150

Gay and lesbian issues
- The **Lesbian and Gay Equality Project (OUT)** offers support and counselling to the gay and lesbian community: Pretoria 012 344 6501; Johannesburg 011 487 3810
- The **Triangle Project** offers support and counselling to the gay and lesbian community: Cape Town 021 448 3812. The Zimbabwean equivalent is: **GALZ**, 35 Colenbrander Road, Milton Park, Harare: (04) 706531

Legal and related advice
- **Legal Aid** offers legal advice and assistance: Cape Town 021 6965172; Johannesburg 011 8772000. Consult your local telephone directory for a number close to you
- **Tshwaranang Advocacy Centre** offers legal advice, including to victims domestic violence: Johannesburg 011-4034267

Pregnancy and abortion
- **Mary Stopes Clinic** does termination of unwanted pregnancies and offers advice and counselling: Tollfree 0800 117785
- **Love in Action** offers support during pregnancy: Cape Town 021 376 1440
- **Safe Line** is a helpline offering support to victims of teenage pregnancy: Tollfree 0800 035 553

Rape
- **Rape Crisis** offers counselling, support and advice to rape victims. They have call centres in most cities and some big towns. Consult your local telephone directory for the number closest to you.

www.ingramcontent.com/pod-product-compliance
Lightning Source LLC
Chambersburg PA
CBHW072154270326
41930CB00011B/2416